THE SCIENTI-FIT

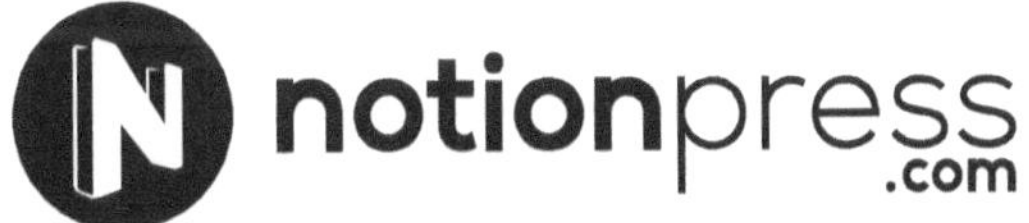

THE SCIENTI-FIT

LOGICAL FITNESS THROUGH THE EYES OF A HEART SURGEON

DR. KALPESH MALIK

Senior Cardio-Vascular and Thoracic Surgeon

IFBB certified Bodybuilders' and Master Trainer

ISSA certified Sports Nutritionist

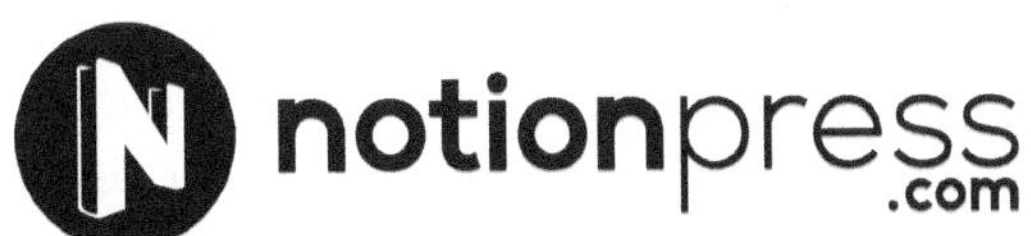

Notion Press

Old No. 38, New No. 6
McNichols Road, Chetpet
Chennai - 600 031

First Published by Notion Press 2017
Copyright © Dr. Kalpesh Malik 2017
All Rights Reserved.

ISBN 978-1-947498-46-4

This book is a tribute to MIKE MENTZER, one of the greatest bodybuilders of all times, a rare combination of brain and brawn, whose thinking and philosophy paved the way for my concept of logical medical practice and fitness. His writings and ideas inspired me to always think logically and never compromise on my principles in life and do what I think is best for my patients and fitness clients.

– Dr. Kalpesh Malik.

CONTENTS

PREFACE

WHY DID I WRITE THIS BOOK?

I am Dr. Kalpesh Malik, a practising Consultant Cardiac Surgeon since 2000 A.D. I deal with the heart and all its problems. I have been associated with thousands of Cardiac Surgeries since then and I have personally operated more than 7500 cardiac surgeries till date. I have been hearing many words since decades like 'Good Cholesterol,' 'Bad Cholesterol,' 'Serum Lipids' and many others day in and day out. These words form a part of my daily language, but, they have failed to convince me as regarding their authenticity. I have been questioning their validity since a long time.

As I dealt with more and more patients, certain realisations dawned on me:

(1) Not all Coronary Heart diseases have Cholesterol as their root cause. In fact, I have seen prescriptions of the 'so called Cholesterol Lowering agents' prescribed even for normal blood cholesterol levels.

(2) If more than 90% of your body's cholesterol is synthesized by your own body (liver, kidneys, many hormone producing glands etc.), how can it be harmful?

(3) For management of diseases and also their prevention, medications are not the only answer. A good customised diet plan plus a proper exercise regimen suiting an individual's health and fitness goals works wonders for the health and can bring down the requirements of medicines, most of which might not even be required at a later stage.

(4) Diabetes type II, Hypertension (high BP), Osteoporosis (weak bones in old age) as well as Osteoarthritis are lifestyle related

ailments. A change in the lifestyle along with a proper nutritious diet and a proper exercise prescription can prevent, control or sometimes even reverse these diseases.

(5) All the doctors say that prevention is better than cure. But, how much time and money is being spent on prevention? Practically, nothing! Preventive Health check-ups done in the name of prevention are merely aids to early diagnosis of a disease, but they do not do anything for preventing these diseases. Prevention starts at a very early age, much before the appearance of these diseases.

(6) Most of the cardiac patients who have undergone angioplasty or bypass surgery are scared to venture back to a normal lifestyle. It is my endeavour that every cardiac patient should be living a healthy life full of vitality and vigour.

These observations are merely glimpses into the fallacies in the medical field. Let's now talk about the fitness and the wellness industry. I have been into fitness since a long time, longer than I can remember. Like most people, I also thought that performing a certain set of exercises daily can make me achieve the physique of my dreams. I used to exercise daily and simultaneously consume huge amounts of proteins, carbohydrates and fats. I also used to eat a lot of junk foods thinking that as I was exercising vigorously, most of this food was feeding my muscles. I gradually experienced a significant increase in my strength, but, simultaneously I also gained a huge amount of fat. My peers and friends used to appreciate the huge size of my arms, but at the same time, also used to poke fun at my huge belly. Mind you, the size of my waist three years back used to be 37 inches (now it has shrunk to a mere 28 inches). One fine day, I started to wonder where I was going wrong. I was very strong in mathematics and chemistry in my school days. Biochemistry of the human body (biochemistry deals with the chemical composition of the human body as well as the chemical reactions which take place to keep the human body in a running condition) was one of my strongest subjects in Medical College. I realised that if I have to lose body fat quantitatively that is losing certain kilograms of body fat, I should be eating a set amount of calories with the carbohydrates, proteins and fats in a particular ratio which suits my body. That is when I put my thoughts into action. The next thing I did was to start studying again and did these two certifications:-

(1) Diploma in SPORTS NUTRITION from INTERNATIONAL SPORTS SCIENCES ASSOCIATION, CA.

(2) ADVANCED BODYBUILDER'S TRAINER AND MASTER TRAINER COURSE from INTERNATIONAL FEDERATION OF BODYBUILDING.

After acquiring these two diplomas, I hit upon the idea of 'QUANTIFIED NUTRITION.' Eating the correct ratio of carbohydrates, proteins and fats and in particular quantities according to your body's needs can rapidly bring about your body's transformation. WE ARE WHAT WE EAT. Also, the exercises prescribed should go hand in hand with the diet prescribed to an individual. I also brought in all the principles which I had learnt in my Medical College as well as my experience of 28 years in medicine. Here again, I would like to emphasize these very important points:

(1) The day I joined these two diploma courses in fitness, I realised that doctors and dieticians have a very poor knowledge regarding nutrition and exercise physiology. I was no exception before. But, after finishing these two diplomas, my knowledge felt complete and I was able to manage my patients in a much better way.

(2) There are scores of 'half-baked dieticians' in the market who give you a pre-formed diet and charge you a huge packet. They can tell you that a certain food is rich in carbohydrates or proteins or fats, but I have yet to see a dietician who can tell you the exact amount of these macronutrients in a particular food.

(3) Since childhood, we have been imbibed with the knowledge that fats are bad for health. I say that even excess carbohydrates or proteins are bad for health. By the word 'excess,' I mean those quantities which are more than your daily requirements. NOT ALL FATS ARE BAD IF TAKEN IN THE RIGHT PROPORTIONS.

(4) METABOLISM: This word means the ability of the body to burn calories to maintain its functions. Metabolism is dependent upon three things:

- ✦ Your daily activity level.
- ✦ Your fat free lean body mass.
- ✦ Your hormones.

Through QUANTIFIED DIETS and proper insertion of appropriate exercises in your daily schedule, each of these factors can be modified to suit your goals.

Also, since I have been intimately associated with gymnasiums and trainers and all sorts of supplements, I have been able to accurately pinpoint what are the shortcomings in the fitness world. Let me try to explain this to you by the following points:

(1) Most of the trainers in the gyms are non-certified. They learn from their seniors who are themselves non-certified. We call it 'BROSCIENCE.' Most of their efforts at making you fit are a 'Hit-or-miss affair.' They might succeed or they might not. Usually, they don't succeed. Some of them are certified trainers but, their studies have been directed only towards the techniques of the exercises. They are unaware of either the anthropometry of the human body, the hormonal changes happening in the body at the time of exercise and afterwards or the nutritional aspects of fitness. Many of them are steroid users and they lure their clients towards using the 'gear.' They are unaware of the illegitimacy of steroids, the complications of using steroids in bodybuilding and how to monitor and tackle the side effects of steroids. Ultimately, the damage done is to their clients only which is usually irreversible.

(2) Most of the dieticians we find in the gyms are not well versed in the field of fitness nutrition or sports nutrition. As a result, they are not aware of the concept of 'Quantified nutrition' or 'customized diet plans.' Every human being is unique as regarding height, weight, age, body fat percentage, daily activities, food preferences and timings etc. The diet should be tailor-made for

each client and should never be a general diet applicable to all. It never works. Many of them copy the diet plans available on the internet with all the exotic food items like fillet, tuna, salmon, quinoa etc. The list is endless. I bet many of them must not even have seen these food items.

(3) Most of the diets prescribed by dieticians pertain to weight loss. The dieticians fail to understand the difference between weight loss and fat loss. These diets usually cause water loss initially followed by muscle loss and if you are very lucky, then some fat loss as well.

(4) The trainers or the dieticians try to sell you supplements. There are various supplements available in the market like protein powders, creatine powders, BCAA, glutamine, CLA etc. The list is endless. They tell you that these supplements will give you the desired body of your dreams. The word 'SUPPLEMENT' means that it is a supplement to the diet taken. Diet forms the main bulk of the nutritional aspect of fitness and supplements are just additives in case you need them. They can never replace a good diet.

(5) Many of the exercise regimens prescribed to you in the gymnasiums are taken from bodybuilding magazines and the internet. Many of us surf the internet and copy the workout schedules of our favourite bodybuilders. But, we are all unaware of the story behind the scenes and that is almost all the bodybuilders are on high doses of anabolic steroids. With anabolic steroids, the recovery after exercise is faster. The muscle growth is much more. If you are a natural athlete that is if you have never touched these steroids and don't want to touch them now or ever, just remember one thing: These workout schedules are not for you.

Through this book, it is my endeavour to bring to you the correct fundamentals of medicine, nutrition and exercise. I would like to summarise my successful experiences both on myself and more than 1200 clients of mine, and I am proud to announce that the transformation rate of my clients is nearly 100%. The principles are:

(1) Nutrition is 'quantified.'

(2) Go for 'Fat loss,' not 'weight loss.'

(3) Body weight is not important. Body composition is important. When you exercise and diet correctly, you build muscles and also lose a significant amount of fat. Since muscles are heavier than fat, you might end up weighing more than your initial weight, but your mirror will tell you that you look leaner.

(4) As your body composition changes with diet and exercise, so does your metabolism and your hormones. You will look younger and feel younger. You will undergo an 'Age reversal.'

(5) You need not spend hours in the gym daily to achieve your dream physique. Half hour workouts three times a week is more than enough to achieve your top fitness level. But then, exercise schedules cannot be generalised. Each person is unique and his/her needs are different.

(6) You don't need all the supplements available in the market to achieve your dream physique. If you can acquire all the nutrients you need from your diet itself, you won't need supplements. Only if because of certain food preferences, you are unable to meet your nutritional requirements, then and then only you should go for supplements. But, as I said, it purely depends on your needs and goals. If you are a bodybuilder or a top level athlete, you might need supplements. Please note that I used the words 'MIGHT NEED,' not 'WILL NEED.'

Let us now move on to sports. I have categorized physical sports mainly into three types:

(1) Power Sports, such as weight lifting, power lifting, shot put throw, discus throw, javelin throw, high jump etc.

(2) Endurance sports which need stamina such as marathons, long distance cycling, long distance swimming, triathlons etc.

(3) Combination of the above like tennis, football, hockey etc.

You can see that each of these sports are very different in nature. Their intensities are different, their durations are different and hence, their training and nutritional requirements have to be different. It will be my endeavour through this book to guide you towards these fundamentals in their correct light.

These are my aims in writing this book. Let us all navigate towards our correct understanding of the fitness principles so as to live a fitter life and stay away or even reverse all the lifestyle ailments like diabetes type II, hypertension, cardiac diseases, osteoporosis, osteoarthritis and many others. Also, it will be my effort to explain to you that these diseases cannot and should not be a hindrance for you in living your life to its fullest potential.

So, no more excuses! Let's all be 'SCIENTIFITS.'

ACKNOWLEDGEMENTS

I feel a deep gratitude and love for my wife Ravinder Kaur who inspired me towards fitness and whose persistent dedication and efforts drove me towards writing this book. Here, I would definitely mention my son Armaan Malik, without whose loving distractions, this book would have been written in half the time.

I am greatly indebted to the thousands of my patients and their families who expressed their full faith in me and submitted themselves to my care. I also express my heartiest thanks to all my fitness clients for giving me an opportunity to transform themselves and their lives.

I take this opportunity to appreciate the efforts of those scores of trainers who helped my clients in achieving their fitness goals.

– Dr. Kalpesh Malik.

CHAPTER 1

WHAT IS FITNESS?

Let's take an arbitrary scenario. There is a certain person who is slim with less fat on his/her body. Now, that does not mean that the fat percentage is low. It merely indicates that the person is slim. This person does not smoke or drink alcohol. He/she sleeps for 8 hours in the night. Only thing that is missing is that this person does not exercise or does not eat the right kind of diet. But, at the same time this person does not have any of the lifestyle related diseases. Let us assume that this person lives on the 4th floor of an apartment building and one fine day the lift is not working and this particular person has to climb the stairs. By the time he/she reaches the required floor, he/she is literally steaming and huffing and puffing. The heart rate is elevated and the blood pressure is shooting through the roof. The clothes are drenched in sweat and the person is breathless. Is the person fit?

Let's take a look at another scenario. We have a person who is young, lean and muscular. He exercises in the gym daily and eats a clean meal most of the time. By the word, 'clean' I mean that he avoids junk food and never over eats. He has shirt-rippling muscles and has that classy figure which makes women look at him in sheer admiration and men in sheer envy. Now, suppose this person goes to a supermarket and it so happens that he has to carry heavy grocery bags to his home which is half a kilometre away. He looks furtively here and there for a conveyance and he finds none. This same person who lifts insane amounts of weights in the gym cannot carry grocery bags which are not even half the weight what he throws in the gym. Would you call him fit?

So, what is fitness?

According to the Centre for Disease Control and Prevention (CDC), physical fitness is defined as the ability to carry out daily tasks with vigour and alertness, without undue fatigue, and with ample energy to enjoy leisure time pursuits and also respond to emergencies.

Let us now elaborate this definition in detail.

Every individual is different in a way that every individual has his/her own lifestyle, occupation and daily activity level. The amount of physical activity done for the daily tasks of each individual is different. Imagine a CEO of a company who primarily has a desk job. Compare this person to a surgeon who has to stand for long hours in the operation theatre and also has to move about the hospital. The third person is a construction site worker. Now, the daily physical activity of each of these three people is different. So will be their energy requirements and their stamina. A construction worker has much more physical stamina than the CEO. For him, working for long hours at the construction site and lifting heavy weights and drilling and climbing up the scaffolding comprise his daily activity. I am sure that the CEO or the surgeon might not be able to carry out these tasks with ease. For them, this will translate into a very heavy exercise for which their bodies are unaccustomed. Their body will see this as a great stress, whereas for the worker, this is normal routine work. The ability to carry out their daily respective activities with ease comprises one aspect of fitness.

The other aspect of fitness is having an ample reserve energy after the expenditure incurred on performing their daily routine activities. Imagine that the CEO comes home and his son wants to play football with him. Same scenario is with the surgeon and the construction site worker. Don't you think that the fitness level of each of these three persons needs to be different to carry out even these extra activities with ease?

Now, the third aspect of the equation is dealing with emergencies. What is meant by the word emergency is 'Unaccustomed Exercise.' This can be of any form. The CEO might be living on the 10th floor of the apartment building and one fine day, if the lift stops working and he has to climb all the way to his apartment, this comprises an emergency for him. The surgeon when he gets a bus full of trauma casualties and he has to run from pillar to post to manage these patients comes as an emergency to him. Emergency for the construction worker is much more rigorous. Construction sites are known to collapse. Imagine the physical activity involved in evacuating people trapped under the debris. Wouldn't this comprise a tremendous amount of unaccustomed exercise for the worker?

The definition of fitness means that when a person in his/her own sphere of activity can perform his/her daily routine activity as well as leisure activities and still has reserve energy available to perform unaccustomed exercise, then and then only the person is called fit.

Fitness does not mean that the person has to go to the gym daily and lift heavy weights and has to diet like a prisoner of war or has to deny oneself the pleasures of life like going out with friends once in a while and enjoy a bottle of beer. Fitness also does not mean eating only certain foods cooked in certain oils with the tall claims that they protect the heart and are good for the well-being of an individual. Fitness involves a much more holistic approach in that there are multiple approaches to fitness.

It is a much more scientific discipline than merely surfing the internet and blindly following the advices of the so-called half-baked fitness gurus who themselves resort to the internet for their knowledge.

So, why do we need fitness when we have a thriving medical industry?

We have looked at the above scenarios in great detail. Fitness is an integral part of staying healthy. You have an abundance of energy. You have the stamina to carry out whatever tasks are given to you from morning till night. Almost all of us feel fatigued at the end of the day. Just imagine that even at this time, you are feeling bright and chirpy. You come home full of vitality and vigour and spend quality time with your family. You have time and energy to hang out with your friends even when the day has taken its toll. For the workaholics, you still have the mental alertness to have late night meetings where you can discuss business at ease. Isn't that what all of us want?

Looking from the medical point of view, various lifestyle ailments have cropped up like diabetes mellitus type II, hypertension, depression, cardiac problems to name a few. It is very convenient for the medical industry to blame it on stress, but is it really stress that is taking its toll? I don't think so. It is our tendency not to give time to ourselves and not to take the commitment of being fit. We all seek the easy way out. Fast foods have come in the market. Previously, only burgers or pizzas were available. Now, as if that is not enough, these outlets give out various combinations, what they call 'combos' of French fries, fried chips and soft drinks along with the burgers and pizzas. We are addicted to this lifestyle. Who is going to take pains to prepare a healthy meal at home when it is much more convenient to go through the 'drive thru' and collect these combos? This is a jet age. Everyone wants instant gratification.

The abundance of luxuries available at a price, of course, has led all of us into the rat race. Everyone wants a few bucks more so that they can buy these items more and more. Working overtime and doing extra jobs to make the extra buck leaves us very little time to exercise and plan our meals. So, we resort to fast food. These fast food chains give delivery at home or at the workplace. Munching on these foods while working can make you eat much more than what you really need. We overeat, we do not exercise and we blame it on stress. Again, a matter of convenience, isn't it!

This kind of sedentary or physically underactive lifestyle, eating unhealthy foods and lack of rest are the three pillars on which the lifestyle maladies like obesity, diabetes, hypertension, and coronary artery diseases are built. And they are the very pillars which need to be shaken, broken and rebuilt so that fitness can be achieved. I will elaborate it in the subsequent chapters.

Think logical. Act logical.

Be SCIENTIFIT!

CHAPTER 2

WHY PEOPLE SPEND MORE MONEY ON ILLNESS THAN WELLNESS AND FITNESS?

THERE IS A BIG DIFFERENCE BETWEEN HEALTH AND THE MEDICAL INDUSTRY.

Sickness industry services (hospitals, pharma companies and doctors) seek to either treat the symptoms of diseases or eliminate the diseases rather than preventing them. Whereas fitness and wellness industry provides services to healthy people or people having lifestyle diseases like diabetes type II, hypertension etc. to make them feel and look even healthier, to slow the effects of ageing and/or to prevent lifestyle diseases from developing in the first place. The entire sickness or medical industry is so focussed on managing diseases that prevention has taken a back seat altogether. Screening tests as part of health packages that are done in the name of prevention are always aimed at early diagnosis of the diseases rather than their prevention.

Private sector hospitals nowadays are more like five star hotels. And let's be honest for once. No one opens a hospital to give service to the poor. Service to humanity is a by-product and not the main motto, though every such organization says otherwise. Each is concerned with profit. The health sector gives employment to thousands of doctors, paramedical and other auxiliary staff. If the hospital has to employ doctors and other staff of the highest quality, then it costs money and truckloads of it. State of the art medical equipments cost money. There is a race between every hospital to provide luxuries like five star rooms, five star cafeterias, central air conditioning, round the clock ambulance services and other services. And over and above that, these services have to be sustainable and profitable. Don't you think it is more profitable for the sickness industry to manage and treat diseases rather than prevent them? Most of their propaganda is directed towards designing various treatment options for diseases. These options are costly, but not necessarily more effective. In the midst of all this whirlwind, why should anyone bother about prevention? After all, who wants to incur losses?

Look at the Food Industry, which also spends crores on advertisements of their food products, most of which are junk foods. Let's take an instance of fat free foods. These foods are loaded with carbohydrates and sugars to make them tastier. Where do you think these excess sugars go in your body? Obviously to your fat depots! They are more harmful than the original products which might have been containing some amounts of fats. But, look at their advertisements. They are so catchy that people flock to the fat free food counters in hordes. And the result is that Obesity is on the rise in spite of these fat free products which practically run the food markets now. Ironical, isn't it!

Many misleading advertisements are put up but, who bothers! All of us are slaves of the gustatory sensation, meaning taste. Recently, one advertisement is on a rampage in all the newspapers, television and radio channels that food cooked in a particular vegetable oil brings down blood sugars and controls your diabetes. The advertisement runs as "Ab sugars par control karo, khane par nahin." What absolute absurdity, what absolute nonsense! But, neither the government cares about such false propaganda, nor the public. And it is not surprising that sales of that particular cooking oil has gone up.

Should we look at the Pharma industry now? The myth of cholesterol as the root cause of coronary heart disease has been so deeply rooted in the minds of the people by all the calculated advertisements of the pharma industry that it has become a very hard thing to convince the public that there is no such connection. These companies through various channels have properly decimated the market and made it submissive to their directives. Then, they send their very eloquent sales representatives to the over-worked doctors who are extremely busy to question anything. These doctors are bombarded with pamphlets and brochures depicting various pseudo-research studies sponsored by these same pharma companies, and that's another very major and effective channel by which this misinformation is passed onto the consumers (in this case, patients).

Now, who do you think will benefit from the immense profits made by the pharma companies and the food industry? Much of the information that is presented to the government by the Health policy makers is totally outdated. The multi-billion dollar food and pharma industries sponsor many of the health projects of the government. Hence, they get away with any kind of nonsense advertisements which turn the minds of people more towards sickness than health and wellness.

It is very obvious from the above discussions why the Insurance companies don't give any provisions for claims on expenditure incurred for any fitness and wellness programs.

Now, let's view the problem from the perspective of the consumer. Why do you think anyone will spend on disease prevention? People think that if the disease has not happened till now, it might never happen. Why spend money on an uncertain future? And fitness involves a complete change in their lifestyle, something that they are used to since childhood. And a change in the lifestyle to remain fit has to be a permanent change. It requires a lot of determination, dedication and discipline. It also requires a lot of physical activity which most of us shun to do. So, people hesitate to spend money on fitness. If the disease occurs, and the patient spends money, the patient feels that the money has been spent on a just cause and for a proper reason.

All of us are to blame. It is high time that the public reconsiders its position on fitness and wellness. Remember, you might be healthy now but, it is an indisputable fact that your body is slowly ageing and killing itself. You never know what diseases might be developing in your body. Don't wait for them to develop. Prevent them. Live a healthy lifestyle. Exercise hard and eat right. You will develop energy levels you never even dreamt before.

CHAPTER 3

PALLIATIVE SUPERSPECIALISATION

ALMOST ALL DISEASES MANAGED BY SUPER SPECIALISTS
HAVE PALLIATION AS THEIR END TREATMENT AND ARE
MOSTLY PREVENTABLE BY PROPER NUTRITION AND
PHYSICAL EXERCISE.

There are three different terms used by doctors to describe how a disease is handled by them:

(1) Treatment: Some diseases have a definite underlying cause that can be treated. For example, malaria is caused by P. Vivax parasite. There is a definite cure for this disease in the form of drugs such as Chloroquine, Primaquine, Artemisinin etc.

(2) Managing diseases like diabetes type II, hypertension, migrane and almost all the diseases whose definite cause is not known. All that is done is just trying to control the clinical manifestations of the disease like bringing down the blood sugars or decreasing blood pressure. According to the medical fraternity, no cure exists for such diseases. We conveniently call them 'Idiopathic' and blame them on heredity and genetics.

(3) Palliation: Palliation means decreasing the severity of the disease by various interventions. For example, a patient comes with a heart attack. An artery supplying the particular area of the heart is blocked. The cardiologist performs an emergency Angioplasty and Stenting of the artery. The artery opens up and the symptoms of heart attack decrease. But, the root cause behind the heart attack that is the tendency of the body to cause blockages in the arteries is still present. The cardiologist has merely restored the blood supply to the heart muscle. This is palliation, not treatment.

Palliation in super specialisation

Nearly all the diseases managed by super specialists have palliation as their main management. I have given you an example of a cardiologist opening up an artery. Let us take another example. A patient comes with multiple blockages in all the arteries supplying the heart. A cardiac surgeon performs a Bypass operation in this patient. The very meaning of the word 'Bypass' means he/she merely bypasses the blocked segment of the artery using the arteries or the veins of the patient's own body. It is like a busy cross road having a perpetual traffic jam wherein the authorities decide to make a fly over bypassing the area or a main water line which is completely choked up and a plumber makes an alternative channel for the flow of water bypassing the blocked area. Do you get the similarities? All said and done, the primary reason why the blockage happened is still there and it can again cause re-blockages. I can give you an endless list of examples like these. A Nephrologist manages a patient of kidney failure by medicines first, then by dialysis and if conditions permit, a kidney transplant. But, understand that the Nephrologist does not have the means to reverse a kidney back to health which has already failed. The main cause still lurks in the body. Imagine a Gastro-enterologist managing a case of jaundice. Some cases like Jaundice due to stones in the gall bladder and the bile duct (the tube draining bile in the intestines) can be managed by removing the stones, but, that is not a guarantee that these stones will never re-occur. A neurosurgeon removes a tumour from the brain, but, is it a guarantee that this tumour will not reform? Or an Oncologist removing a cancer from the body is not a safe guarantee that now, the cancer will not reoccur.

I am not saying that all of these ailments which require only their clinical manifestations to be managed or palliated by super specialist doctors are preventable by proper nutrition or exercise, but yes, I am definitely saying that a good deal of them can be definitely avoided.

CHAPTER 4

FITNESS AS A WHOLE

As we saw in the previous chapter, there are three main pillars of fitness:

(1) Active lifestyle and Physical exercise.

(2) Correct nutrition.

(3) Rest.

I have been asked many times by people that what is the contribution of each of these to fitness in terms of percentages. I say that each of these need to be carried out to 100% if you want to achieve results.

Active lifestyle and physical exercise

This comprises the first pillar of fitness. Exercise has many benefits, some of which are enumerated below:-

- ✧ Body when subjected to increasing levels of unaccustomed exercise adapts by increasing its strength and flexibility.

- ✧ Muscles grow in size. The bones, cartilages, ligaments and tendons become stronger.

- ✧ Muscle contraction becomes more efficient and progressively uses lesser energy to lift heavier weights.

- ✧ Metabolism of the body receives a boost. Metabolism means the chemical processes that take place in the body of an individual in order to sustain life. Increase in metabolism leads to the body spending more and more energy even at rest and hence, there is lesser chance of the individual getting fat.

- ✧ The system of blood supply in the body comprises the heart, arteries and veins. Exercise keeps this system functioning smoothly with an unhampered blood flow. There is less chance of developing blockages in these arteries. The incidence of cardiac diseases and stroke decreases dramatically with exercise.

- ✧ Exercise tends to give you an energy boost. You feel refreshed the whole day and experience an abundance of energy.

- ✧ Exercise keeps the hormones of the body functioning smoothly. It prevents or delays the onset of lifestyle maladies like diabetes, hypertension etc.

- ✧ Exercise makes you sleep better. The quantity and quality of sleep improves.

- ✧ Rigorous exercise leads to an endorphin surge in the brain. Endorphins are chemicals secreted in the brain which are mood elevators. Happiness levels increase dramatically.

- ✧ Exercise gives you a good physique. This leads to increased self-confidence which translates into success in all aspects of life like business, relationships etc.

- ✧ A person learns to set and achieve goals in life.

Exercise can be aerobic or anaerobic. Aerobic is a less intense type of exercise. We all use oxygen to maintain life. During exercise, the requirement of oxygen increases manifold. The body tries to keep up with this increased demand in form of increased rate of breathing and increased volume of breath intake. If this compensatory mechanism of the body is able to keep up with the oxygen requirement, this is referred to as aerobic exercise. Jogging, dancing or Zumba are forms of aerobic exercise.

Now, let us throw some light on anaerobic exercise. When the body's oxygen intake is unable to meet the increased demand of oxygen during exercise, we call it anaerobic exercise. Weight training is one form of anaerobic exercise. Lifting very heavy weights or sprinting at your near maximum speed imposes a much greater demand of oxygen on the body than can be instantly met.

A judicious combination of aerobic and anaerobic exercise will lead to overall fitness as will be discussed subsequently.

Correct nutrition

It is inconceivable to think of fitness without nutrition. Nutrition is the most important pillar of fitness. You cannot out-run a bad diet. When you are exercising, you need increased calories and the right ratios of carbohydrates, proteins and fats. The body also needs the correct amounts of micronutrients like vitamins and minerals. Precise and quantified nutrition is the key.

Rest

This is the most disregarded but, an equally important pillar of fitness. When you are exercising, your body undergoes something known as 'stress.' Your heart rate increases, your breathing increases, your blood pressure increases etc. Many such changes happen in the body. During intense weight training, many small micro tears happen in the exercising muscles. The tendons are placed under tension and the ligaments of the joints are stretched. All these need to heal in a stronger way for the strength to increase. Also, many hormonal changes happen in the body for the anabolic response to happen. Anabolism is the recovery and growth phase of the body. A deep sleep refreshes your body and your mind so that you are ready for the next day. A small 'power nap' in the afternoon works wonders for your mental alertness.

ACT SCIENTIFIT!

CHAPTER 5

AN OVERVIEW OF THE BASICS OF NUTRITION

The search for foods that enhance performance dates back thousands of years. Warriors used to be fed on high protein diets so as to increase their fighting skills. But, the scientific concepts of nutrition have come into picture quite recently. Understanding the concept of macronutrients and micronutrients and their requirements for different individuals and different sports has led to formulation of diets that not only promote fitness, but also maximise athletic performance. 'Glycogen super compensation' is one such concept which has revolutionised endurance sports. This concept is also applicable in bodybuilding in the pre competition stage, though in a slightly modified form.

The macronutrients

Macronutrients like carbohydrates, proteins, fats and water are needed daily by the body and are measured in grams or litres. Each individual is different as regards his/her body habitus and hence, the requirements of each of them for each of us is very different. I will explain them in detail in the subsequent chapters. I will briefly summarise each of them here.

Carbohydrate is like the high-octane fuel for the body. It is a source of instant energy. Brain primarily utilises glucose as the fuel. Carbohydrates are stored in the muscles and liver. The liver maintains blood glucose levels. Each gram of carbohydrate yields 4 kcal.

Proteins are building blocks of the body. Almost every organ will be having protein as its main brick and mortar. Proteins are also used as enzymes which serve as catalysts (catalysts are the chemicals which speed up other chemical reactions in the body) and also serve as neurotransmitters (chemicals which transmit the current from the brain to the skeletal muscles). Some of the important hormones are proteins which are responsible for growth. Proteins are used in abundance by athletes and bodybuilders because it increases performance. Each gram of protein yields 4 kcal.

Fat is the third most important macronutrient. It along with proteins forms the building blocks of all the body's tissues. It acts as a reservoir of energy. Many hormones are made up of a type of fat known as Cholesterol. Fat soluble vitamins like A, D and E are absorbed along with fat. Each gram of fat yields 9 kcal. of energy. This calorie yield is the highest for any macronutrient.

Water is the fourth macronutrient and a very essential one. 65% of the body weight comprises of water. All the chemical reactions take place in water. Blood which is the nectar of life is composed of almost 80% of water and is essential for transporting nutrients to the tissues and disposal of waste products which are the result of tissue breakdown and residues of chemical reactions. It transports oxygen from the lungs and carbon dioxide to the lungs. One needs to drink water in litres to have optimum health.

Oxygen is the elixir of life. It is inhaled as air by the lungs and transported to the tissues by blood. It is used in oxidisation of fuels like carbohydrates, fats and proteins. This oxidation generates a chemical compound known as adenosine triphosphate (ATP) which is the energy currency of the body. Body utilises energy via ATP. Aerobic training if done judiciously will lead to increased lung capacity and increased tendency of the lungs to absorb oxygen. This translates into better fuel combustion and oxidation and more ATP formation. Performance improves. Oxygen has a dark side also in that it causes oxidative damage of tissue chemicals by formation of toxic free radicals (these will be explained in detail in later chapters). This oxidative damage is responsible for ageing and various diseases like coronary artery disease, arthritis, dementia, diabetes type II, hypertension and even cancer. So, the substance which gives life has the quality to take away life if taken in excess.

Whether Alcohol should or should not be included in the list of macronutrients is left up to the readers. It is a recreational substance but, is also used in many pharmaceutical syrups. It yields 7 kcal. per gram. Apart from its caloric value, use of alcohol inhibits fat and carbohydrate metabolism and thus, is indirectly associated with obesity.

The micronutrients

Micronutrients are substances required by the body in minute quantities like milligrams or micrograms. Vitamins and minerals fall into this category. Vitamins are of two types: fat soluble like Vitamin A, D and E and water soluble like Vitamin B complex and Vitamin C. They serve as catalysts in many chemical reactions. Catalysts serve as boosters of chemical reactions in the body. Many chemical reactions cannot happen in absence of vitamins. To achieve a high level of fitness, the doses of vitamins have to exceed far beyond what is prescribed in RDAs. I will explain about the RDAs in the subsequent paragraphs.

Minerals are very essential to survival. Sodium, Chlorine and Potassium maintain the water balance in the body. Calcium acts as a structural unit of bone. Iron is found in haemoglobin which transports oxygen in the blood. Iodine is used in thyroid hormones production. Chromium is used for the action of Insulin hormone. Zinc is used in tissue healing and for the formation of the male hormone testosterone. Various other minerals like selenium, magnesium, boron, germanium etc. are used in the body in various chemical reactions. So, it is very apparent that micronutrients are as important as macronutrients in the daily diet.

RDA (Recommended Daily Allowances)

The RDAs were first established in 1943 by the US government as "Essential Nutrition to survival." You must have seen the word RDA printed on many food labels. RDA caters to the general population and is primarily concerned with disease prevention resulting from deficiencies of essential nutrients. But, the quantities of nutrients required for achieving optimum health is much more than what is recommended in the RDAs. The most common example is the wide spread general belief that proteins should be taken in quantities of 0.7 to 1.0 grams per kilogram body weight. This quantity might be adequate for survival but, it is in no way adequate for achieving optimum health and absolutely inadequate for optimum athletic performance. So, the next time your doctor tells you that 60 grams proteins per day is adequate for you, question the doctor.

Bioavailability

Bioavailability indicates the amount of nutrient that is absorbed from your digestive tract, from where it enters your blood and is carried to your tissues where it is utilised.

If your diet contains certain nutrients, it does not mean that your body will absorb them and make full use of them. There are many reasons why this happens. Your digestive tract might not be that healthy so that you can absorb the nutrients. For example, there is a chemical in the digestive juices of stomach known as 'Intrinsic factor.' If that is deficient, there is no way that Vitamin B12 can be absorbed. People who are 'lactose intolerant' have problems in digesting milk and milk products. Sometimes, how the nutrients are mixed in food preparations also makes a difference. Presence of calcium in the food retards absorption of zinc. Similarly, calcium and iron together hampers the absorption of iron. The way the food is prepared also makes a huge difference. Too much cooking damages the protein in the food. This is known as denaturation of proteins and it decreases the absorption of proteins.

So, in formulating diet plans, even the question of bioavailability has to be taken into picture. It is not that when a nutritious diet is planned, the work of the nutritionist is over. Substances which do not go together should not be mixed in the same meal. How the food is prepared makes a big difference in how it will ultimately be used by the body. All these factors have to be taken into account in making successful diet plans for the clients.

In the subsequent chapters, we are going to dissect each of the macronutrients and micronutrients in intimate detail relevant to fitness.

EATING THE 'SCIENTI-FIT' WAY!

CHAPTER 6

CARBOHYDRATES: THE HIGH OCTANE FUEL

Carbohydrates are available in a wide variety of sources mainly plants. They are of many kinds:-

(1) Simple Carbohydrates like Glucose, Fructose and Galactose.

(2) Disaccharides are made of two units (molecules) of glucose or one molecule of glucose and one molecule of fructose. There is a third kind of disaccharide called Lactose found in milk which contains one molecule of galactose and one of glucose.

(3) Polysaccharides which are chains of multiple units of glucose. They are also called Complex Carbohydrates. Starch is an example. Another example is Glycogen which is found in animals as the storage form of glucose.

(4) Fibres are made up of carbohydrates called Cellulose. They are found in plants and form the roughage of the diet.

One gram of Glucose gives you 4 kcal. of energy.

Body utilises carbohydrates for instant energy. Brain utilises mainly glucose as fuel. However, in conditions of extreme carbohydrate depletion from the body, the brain may shift towards other fuels like ketones which are derived from fat.

Body utilises both carbohydrates and fats during rest and also, during prolonged endurance kind of activity like marathons. Weight training in fasting state will also utilise both carbohydrates and fats as fuels. However, for intense explosive bursts of activity, the body primarily utilises carbohydrates as fuel.

Many glucose molecules are combined as long chains which are present as starch in plants and glycogen in animals and humans.

Now comes the tricky part of glycogen storage and its effect on the body functions. Glycogen in stored in the body mainly in the liver and skeletal muscles. Brain utilises glucose present in blood. When blood glucose levels go down, liver breaks down glycogen present in it to glucose and this is how, it raises the blood sugar level. Brain functions even when you sleep. Hence, when you wake up in the morning, the liver glycogen stores are usually at a low level. Fruits contain mainly fructose as sugar. Hence, a glass of fruit juice first thing in the morning fills up your liver carbohydrate stores which provides blood glucose which is lapped up by the brain. The reason is that fructose has to pass through the liver first and gets converted to glucose. Liver prefers to fill its stores first. Hence, you feel more refreshed and active after a glass of fruit juice in the morning. But, try going to the gym in the morning drinking only fruit juice. Chances are your workout will suffer that day because fructose does not fill the skeletal muscles' glycogen stores.

On the other hand, glucose and its complex compounds like starch present in the diet will preferentially fill up the muscle glycogen stores and then, the liver stores.

Hormones and their effect on Glucose metabolism

The most essential hormone which regulates blood glucose level is INSULIN which is secreted by a gland known as Pancreas which is situated behind the stomach. When blood glucose levels rise after a meal, insulin gets secreted which drives glucose into body cells. When blood glucose levels fall e.g. after an overnight fast, insulin secretion is shut off. Another hormone known as GLUCAGON is secreted by the pancreas which aids in raising the blood sugar level. Other hormones which help glucagon are stress hormones like Cortisol and Adrenaline. Even Growth Hormone helps in increasing blood sugar levels, though in a weaker way.

Glycemic index and Glycemic load of foods

Certain foods contain carbohydrates in simple forms. These foods get absorbed very rapidly and cause a rapid rise in blood sugar levels. These foods are called 'HIGH GLYCEMIC INDEX FOODS.' Certain foods which contain a large amount of complex carbohydrates take longer time to digest and get absorbed. With these foods, blood sugar levels rise very slowly and remain stable for a longer time. These foods are referred to as 'LOW GLYCEMIC INDEX FOODS.' The glycemic index of foods are compared to glucose which is the simplest and the fastest absorbing sugar and is considered to be having a glycemic index of 100%.

'GLYCEMIC LOAD' is a measure that takes into account the amount of carbohydrates present in a food together with how quickly it will raise the blood sugar level.

Rice, multigrain, sweet potato, yam, kidney beans, chick peas etc. all cause a slow rise in blood sugar levels. They are examples of low glycemic index foods. Sugars and refined flour which are fast absorbing are high glycemic index foods.

Fats if combined with sugars in the diet slow down the absorption of carbohydrates in the preparation. Eating a high fibre diet also slows carbohydrate absorption. These are certain ways how we can decrease the glycemic index of foods.

For the gym fanatics, there is a word of advice. Consume a meal which is containing low glycemic index carbohydrates and some amount of protein about two to three hours prior to an intense exercise session. This will fill up the muscle glycogen stores and your performance will be enhanced. Some people consume high glycemic carbohydrates about an hour prior to exercise. This is the worst thing to do as the increased blood glucose level causes an insulin spike in the body which will lead to a sudden fall in the blood sugar level and your performance in the gym is likely to go down.

Body carbohydrate stores and Glycogen super compensation

The body has limited carbohydrate stores of approximately 400–500 grams. The technique of 'Glycogen Super compensation' also known as 'Carbohydrate loading' works on the principle that when the body's carbohydrate stores are completely depleted and then, filled up, the body can store up to 185% of the muscle's normal carbohydrate storing capacity. This technique of carbohydrate loading is used in various endurance sports and also, as part of pre-contest preparation in bodybuilding.

Fibres

Fibres are polysaccharides which are not digested by the human body. Hence, they do not provide energy. They are made up of carbohydrates like cellulose, hemicellulose, pectin, gums, polysaccharides found in algae etc. They are found in whole grains, fruits especially skin, green leafy vegetables, husk, nuts, seeds etc.

They do not provide energy but, they serve several important functions in the diet. They make up the roughage portion of the diet and aid in the movement of food in the intestines. They make the major bulk of the stools. They delay the gastric emptying and lead to satiety. Fibres in the food slow the absorption of carbohydrates which leads to a slow rise of blood sugar levels. This function is important in diabetics as it leads to better regulation of blood sugar levels.

There is a particular type of water soluble fibre found in oats which is said to decrease the risk of coronary artery disease. This fibre is known as Beta Glucan. It is said that 3 or more grams of Beta Glucan should be present in the diet for this benefit to occur.

For optimum health benefits, fibres should be present in meals in amounts of 40–60 grams.

CHAPTER 7

IS SUGAR A POISON: MY TAKE AGAINST DEMONISATION OF SUGAR!

We all must have come across many people who have practically given up eating table sugar and still, they accumulate a good amount of body fat. There has been a considerable amount of debate about whether sugar is harmful for health or not. I hope this chapter throws some light on the reality.

Sugar is consumed for many centuries in many forms, especially as sweets. It is present as table sugar, cereals and in many types of foods. Fruit juices contain fructose but, the fruit juices that are available in the market have added sugars to make them tastier and preservatives to prolong their shelf lives.

'Is sugar a poison' is a very interesting point of debate. Our society is always on the lookout for 'demons': scapegoats whom they can sacrifice to blanket their misdeeds. In the 1980s, it was 'fats'; now it is 'sugar.'

Let us shift towards more logical thinking. This is what this book is about. Is it really sugar who is the main culprit behind lifestyle diseases like obesity, diabetes type II, hypertension, cardiac diseases and stroke? Or the real reason is something else and we are just trying to find a 'false criminal' who can be sacrificed at the altar, so that our pseudo-conscience remains clear?

Sugar or table sugar, whatever name you give it, is composed of one molecule of glucose and one molecule of fructose. It is split in your digestive tract and absorbed. The glucose portion rapidly enters the blood stream. The fructose portion absorbs poorly, but goes to the liver first. It is converted to glucose by the liver and stored there. Now, if your liver glucose stores are full, this fructose gets converted to glycerol which is the raw material for fat, the very same fat which gets deposited in your body and causes obesity. The glucose in the blood stream causes release of a hormone known as Insulin by your pancreas. This glucose can either be taken up by liver or muscles of the body or it keeps on circulating as blood glucose and is used by the brain for energy.

Now, let us look to the other sources of glucose. All the carbohydrates except fibres are digested into glucose. Glucose is the end product of digestion of any kind of usable carbohydrate. All the foods like rice (both white and brown), oats or the fruits that you eat contain carbohydrates. Once the carbohydrate is digested and the glucose is absorbed, the body cannot distinguish between the glucose that is eaten in any form, be it oats or sugars. Now, think that your body needs 150 grams of carbohydrates per day and you are consuming only healthy carbs but around 200 grams per day, the extra 50 grams will be stored as fat. On the other hand, if your body needs 150 grams of carbohydrates and you are consuming less than that and a few grams of your ingested carbohydrates is sugar, then how can it be harmful? Of course, if your physique is you main source of income e.g. if you are a film actor or a model or a professional bodybuilder, then you take care. But, if you are a common person who is just concerned with fitness, there is no need to deprive yourself of that one teaspoon of sugar which will sweeten your coffee and your day. After all, not all of us are professional physique models or professional bodybuilders, right?

Let us understand this with an example. You consume 10 grams of sugar with your tea. This will contain 5 grams of glucose which is fast-digesting and 5 grams of fructose which is slow digesting. How much damage do you think this will do to your system? I can quote hundreds of food items which have manifold amounts of glucose than your table sugar. Of course, once should try to minimise the hidden sugars present in many items, especially the fat-free foods, but merely shunning that cup of sweet tea just because it contains 5–10 grams of sugar just does not make sense.

There are many lifestyle diseases 'linked' by the media and the medical industry to sugar intake, but is it the only cause of obesity, diabetes, hypertension, cardiac diseases or stroke? I don't think so. Eating excess carbohydrates in any form and a sedentary lifestyle are the root causes. Increased alcohol usage and smoking are other contributory factors. Even excess protein intake is bad. Even drinking massive amounts of water can wreak havoc with your system. True, sugar contains empty calories but, then so are many other food items. Sugar has also been linked to dental caries. It has been suggested that consuming less sugar might have a preventive effect on dental caries. But, it is found that brushing teeth twice daily with a fluoride toothpaste and taking care to maintain a good oral hygiene leads to better improvement in dental caries than merely avoiding sugar.

Your child would be much better off drinking milk with a little cocoa and sugar in it than a glass of sweetened fruit juice. Right or wrong?

My take on sugar is that a little amount, if it fits into you daily recommended carbohydrate intake is not at all harmful. I leave it up to the reader to decide whether sugar is a 'Demon' or not. This topic is open to debate. But, my take on sugar is very clear.

CHAPTER 8

PROTEINS AND AMINO ACIDS: THE BUILDING BLOCKS OF LIFE

In this chapter, I will discuss about proteins and amino acids and their role in the body. I will also clear all the myths regarding the quality and the quantity of proteins in the diet.

The primary role of proteins in the body is to act as building materials for the various body tissues. Also, various hormones and enzymes (they are the catalysts that speed up chemical reactions in the body) are proteins. The brain, spinal cord and the various nerves work by the phenomenon of electrical impulses. Proteins play a very major role in the transmission of impulses along the nerves. Proteins take part in various chemical reactions so essential for sustaining life. They are not the favoured fuel of the body for energy, however during times of starvation or very intense exercise, proteins are broken down to be used as energy.

Proteins are made up of long chains of different chemicals known as 'Amino Acids.' There are 22 amino acids in the body. Some of these cannot be manufactured by our body and should be taken with food. They are known as 'Essential amino acids.' Rest of the amino acids can be synthesized in our body. Hence, they are known as 'Non-essential amino acids.'

Rating the proteins

(1) COMPLETE PROTEINS: They are proteins derived from certain sources that contain all the amino acids that are used by our body, especially the essential amino acids in quantities sufficient for

normal growth and body weight. Usually, proteins derived from animal sources are complete proteins.

(2) INCOMPLETE PROTEINS: They are usually deficient in one or more of the essential amino acids. Plant proteins are usually incomplete.

Proper proportions of all the amino acids, both essential as well as non-essential are necessary for the proteins to be utilised by the body. This is precisely the reason why vegetarian body builders are advised protein supplements, especially those made from milk like Whey and Casein so that the complete profile of amino acids is obtained.

Net Protein Utilisation

Net Protein Utilisation or NPU focuses on digestibility of a protein. It measures the nitrogen intake and output and the amount of protein needed to maintain nitrogen balance. This shows how complete is the digestion of a particular protein. Proteins with high NPU are egg proteins and milk proteins like Whey and Casein. Hence, these are the proteins preferred by athletes and bodybuilders.

Biological value of a protein

Biological value (BV) is a value that is calculated to determine the quality of a protein. It indicates the efficiency with which a protein furnishes the proper amount and proportion of the amino acids needed for synthesis of body proteins i.e. the net utilisation of proteins by the body. In simple words, it indicates the ability of a particular protein to get deposited in tissues so that new tissue proteins are formed. Examples of proteins with high Biological Value is whey, eggs, chicken, meat, fish etc.

It is not prudent to prescribe just any type of protein in the diet. The protein should be prescribed in the correct quantities required by the body taking into account how much will be used by the body and that is determined only by its biological value and how good is your digestion and absorption.

ANABOLISM AND CATABOLISM: The concept of Nitrogen balance

Nitrogen balance is a concept to determine whether the body is in a phase of growth or a phase of decline.

ANABOLISM: This is the growth phase. The body synthesizes new molecules, chemicals and tissues or it strengthens its already existing tissues.

CATABOLISM: This is the reverse of anabolism. The tissues of the body get degraded or broken down.

Now, how does this happen and when does this happen?

It is presumed that body takes in Nitrogen in the form of proteins. Body cannot absorb Nitrogen from the air like oxygen. Hence, the quantity of Nitrogen taken in by a person indirectly reflects the quantity of protein ingested. Proteins are the building blocks of the body. Body is continuously synthesizing new proteins and breaking down old proteins. The amino acids (which are the chemicals which make up proteins) needed for formation of new proteins are obtained either from the breakdown products of the old proteins themselves which are broken down by the body and replaced or the protein taken in the diet. Not all the amino acids in the body are used up for new protein synthesis. Some of them are further broken down in the body to chemicals like urea and expelled through urine, faeces or sweat.

The concept of Nitrogen balance becomes very simple now. If the total amount of nitrogen taken in the diet daily is exactly equal to the total amount of nitrogen lost from the body in urine, faeces or sweat, it means that the body is maintaining its structure as it is; the same amount of new tissue is synthesized as the degrading old tissue and the net tissue amount remains almost the same, the individual is said to be in NITROGEN BALANCE.

If the total amount of nitrogen taken in the food exceeds the nitrogen lost from the body, it means that the body is in an ANABOLIC PHASE that is there is net tissue growth with synthesis of new proteins. The individual is said to be in POSITIVE NITROGEN BALANCE. This happens during puberty, bulking phase of muscle growth, pregnancy, healing from injuries etc. Many anabolic hormones play a very important role in this phase.

If the total amount of nitrogen lost from the body exceeds the amount taken in the diet, it means that more proteins are broken down in the body and less are synthesized. The body is said to be in CATABOLISM (NEGATIVE NITROGEN BALANCE).

Negative nitrogen balance occurs in

- Starvation.
- Fasting for prolonged periods.
- Low calorie diets given by dieticians for fat loss. The amount of proteins in these diets is usually inadequate to meet the body's demands or sometimes, the proteins are in excess and there is very little amount of carbohydrates and fats in the diet. Body then breaks down these proteins and uses them as fuel.
- Severe injuries.
- Severe burns.
- Diseases like Hyperthyroidism, Muscle wasting diseases etc.

HOW TO MEASURE NITROGEN BALANCE

This is performed in the laboratory. Nitrogen content of a food is first measured. Then the nitrogen content of urine, faeces and sweat of that particular individual is measured and nitrogen balance is calculated from these values. This method is very cumbersome and impractical, though very accurate.

HOW DO I DETERMINE NITROGEN BALANCE OF MY CLIENTS

The diets which I prescribe to my clients are quantitative. I know exactly how much protein I am prescribing to a particular client. I ask them to measure their body composition every two weeks. I make a note of the increase in their fat free lean body mass in the body composition.

When I see an increase in their lean body mass, I am satisfied that my clients are in positive nitrogen balance and things are moving in the right direction. A very crude method, but a logical and practical one, don't you agree!

CHAPTER 9

FAT: THE MOST MISUNDERSTOOD MACRONUTRIENT

We have been hammered since childhood about the ill effects of fats. But, the most logical statement is that it is the excess fat which is deposited in the body that is bad and not, the judicious intake of good fats in the diet. In fact, fats make up the highly essential component in our diets. Actually, fat deposits in our body were not at all harmful many centuries ago. At that time, the food was not so plentiful, hence body fat used to be conveniently used as energy during times of food deprivation. As civilisations evolved, the chemical structure of the human body has not changed much and so is its fat storing tendency, but food has become abundant and readily available. Our bodies are not able to use the energy from our fat stores and at the same time, there is a very obvious reason for new fat formation and deposition in the body. Get the picture? A little alteration in your lifestyle and dietary habits can get you lean in no time.

Fats come in various forms collectively known as 'lipids.' Like carbohydrates, lipids are also made of carbon, hydrogen and oxygen atoms. Fats provide maximum number of calories per gram of body weight i.e. 9 kcal per gram.

Let us now extol the virtues of lipids. Some of them are:

(1) As mentioned before, fat deposits act as a huge reservoir of energy. They are supposed to provide our bodies with energy during times of food deprivation.

(2) Lipids are vital for maintaining various body functions. They are important for maintaining the structure and function of the membranes surrounding our cells. Cells make up the units of

body tissues. Body is made up of trillions of cells and fats are very vital for maintaining their structure and function. They help in the transfer of oxygen to the blood in the lungs. They are important for brain and spinal cord function. They play a very major role in many metabolic processes and chemical reactions in the body which are necessary to sustain life. Innumerable such chemical reactions cannot take place without the presence of fats in the body.

(3) Certain essential fatty acids such as Omega 3 & 6 are very important to the body. They reduce blood lipid levels, help against development of Coronary heart diseases and play an important role in body's response to stress. They help in a quicker recovery following stressful exercise.

(4) Fats help in the absorption of fat soluble vitamins like A, D, E & K.

(5) Cholesterol is very important for maintaining integrity of cell membranes, brain and nervous system functions, many chemical reactions and also as raw material for formation of sex hormones like testosterone, estrogen etc.

(6) Fat acts like shock absorber and insulates body organs against injury.

(7) Lipids act as building blocks of various essential biomolecules.

(8) Fats make food very tasty.

(9) Fats are a very important fuel source for endurance athletes like marathoners, long distance swimmers etc.

Saturated fats and unsaturated fats

As I said before, fats are made up of one molecule of Glycerol and three molecules of fatty acids. Further breakdown of the chemical structure reveals fats to be made up of carbon, hydrogen and oxygen. Without going into the intricacies of chemistry, let me give you a broad outline on saturated and unsaturated fats. Saturated fats tend to be more solid at room temperature. Oils are liquid. So, you can easily see from this difference that fats derived from animal sources are usually saturated in nature. Fish have a mixture of saturated and unsaturated fats. Whereas vegetable oils are mainly unsaturated fats. The fatty acids which form the fats can also be classified as short chain fatty acids (if they contain 3–5 carbon atoms), medium chain fatty acids (6–12 carbons), long chain fatty acids (13–19 carbons) and very long chain fatty acids (20 or more carbons). Coconut oil is the only saturated fat which is not solid at room temperature. It contains medium chain fatty acids.

There is another category of fats known as Hydrogenated fats (also known as Trans fats) which are synthesized artificially by passing hydrogen through the vegetable oils under high pressure and temperature in the presence of a catalyst. They tend to be solid at room temperature. Consumption of Trans fats is considered to be bad for health and is linked to various diseases.

Essential fatty acids (Omega 3 & 6)

Almost all the fatty acids can be manufactured by the body with a few exceptions. Two such fatty acids are Linoleic acid (also known as Omega 6) and alpha Linolenic acid (an Omega 3 fatty acid). They are poly-unsaturated fatty acids. It is observed that our diet is rich in Omega 6 fatty acids and low in Omega 3 fatty acids. Furthermore, the consumption of refined sugars, carbohydrates and use of hydrogenated vegetable oils have led to metabolic breakdown in our body and has created a susceptibility towards developing life style diseases.

Recently, Linoleic acid (Omega 6) has been modified into a structure known as CLA (Conjugated Linoleic acid) which is being promoted for its fat burning properties. But, nothing conclusive has been proven yet.

Arachidonic acid is another form of Omega 6 fatty acid formed from Linoleic acid in the body. It plays an important role in the inflammatory reactions of the body (Chemical and physical reactions of the body in response to injury). It also forms an important part of the membrane surrounding the cells.

Alpha-Linolenic acid is an important Omega 3 fatty acid. It forms the raw material for the formation of two other important Omega 3 fatty acids which we all know as EPA and DHA. Both EPA and DHA are also found in cold water fish like cod, salmon, mackerel, sardines, trout and eel. They reduce the inflammatory reactions of the body which might sometimes be harmful, make the blood thin to speed up and smoothen the circulation of blood which results in better oxygen delivery to the tissues, keep blood lipid levels low and prevent heart attacks.

GAMMA LINOLENIC ACID (GLA)

It is another form of Omega 3 fatty acid formed in the body from the Omega 6 fatty acid Linoleic acid. It prevents blood clotting, reduces blood lipid levels, reduces inflammation, improves immunity and regulates handling of calcium by the body. It is found in limited food sources, the major being evening primrose oil, borage oil and black currant oil.

PHOSPHOLIPIDS

Phospholipids are another group of fats containing Phosphorus. They are found in cell membranes and also help in transportation of lipids in the blood. They are important for functioning of the nervous system. A type of Phospholipid known as Choline increases memory and also prevents fat deposits in the liver. We have all heard of fatty liver, right?

CHOLESTEROL

Cholesterol is a form of fat. It is usually synthesized by the body itself. In food sources, it is usually found in non-vegetarian foods like meat, under the skin of chicken, whole milk, eggs and cheese. It is helpful for functioning of the nervous system, takes part in various chemical reactions and is the raw material for formation of hormones like testosterone, oestrogen, stress hormones like cortisol etc.

Cholesterol is finally officially removed from the 'Naughty list'

The US government has finally accepted that 'Cholesterol' is not a nutrient of concern....thus doing a U-turn on their warnings to us to stay away from high cholesterol foods since the 1970s to avoid clogged arteries and heart disease.

This means eggs, butter, full-fat dairy products, nuts, coconut oil and meat have now been classified as 'safe' and have been officially removed from the 'Nutrients of concern' list.

The US department of agriculture, which is responsible for updating the guidelines every five years, stated in its guidelines for 2015: "Previously, the Dietary guidelines for Americans recommended that Cholesterol intake be limited to no more than 300 mg/day. The 2015 DGAC will not bring forward this recommendation because available evidence shows no appreciable relationship between consumption of dietary cholesterol and serum (blood) cholesterol, consistent with the AHA/ACC (American Heart Association/American College of Cardiology). The Dietary Guidelines Advisory Committee will, in response, no longer will warn people against eating high cholesterol foods and will instead focus on sugar as the main substance of dietary concern."

US Cardiologist Dr. Steven Nissen said. "It's the right decision....We got the dietary guidelines wrong...........They've been wrong for decades. When we eat more foods rich in this compound, our bodies make less. If we deprive ourselves of foods high in cholesterol such as eggs, butter, meat, liver etc. our body revs up."

The real truth about Cholesterol

The majority of the Cholesterol in your body is produced by your own liver. It is essential for nerve cells to function. Cholesterol is the base compound for the synthesis of all the steroid hormones including Oestrogen, testosterone and Corticosteroids. HIGH CHOLESTEROL IN THE BODY IS A CLEAR INDICATION WHICH SHOWS THAT THE LIVER OF THE INDIVIDUAL IS IN GOOD HEALTH.

Dr. George V. Mann M.D., associate director of the Framingham study for the Incidence and Prevention of Cardio-Vascular Disease (CVD) and its risk factors states: "Saturated fats and Cholesterol in the diet are not the main cause of coronary heart disease....that myth is the greatest deception of the century, perhaps of any century...........CHOLESTEROL IS THE BIGGEST MEDICAL SCAM OF ALL TIME...............THERE IS NO SUCH THING AS BAD CHOLESTEROL.........

So, you can stop trying to change your Cholesterol level. Studies prove beyond a doubt that Cholesterol doesn't cause heart disease and trying to decrease blood Cholesterol doesn't prevent heart attacks. The majority of people who have heart attacks have normal Cholesterol levels......

OUR BODY NEEDS 950 milligrams OF CHOLESTEROL FOR DAILY METABOLISM AND THE LIVER IS THE MAIN PRODUCER. ONLY 15% OF CHOLESTEROL IS BEING DONATED BY THE FOOD WE EAT..........

If the fat content is less in our food, our liver works more to maintain the level at 950 mg. If the Cholesterol level is high in the body, it shows that the liver is working perfect......

Experts say that there is nothing like LDL or HDL............

Cholesterol is not found to create blockages anywhere in the human body."

AND THE PHARMA AND MEDICAL INDUSTRIES ARE MAKING TRILLIONS OF BUCKS AT YOUR EXPENSE BY PROMOTING WRONG INFORMATION.

CHAPTER 10

SATURATED FATS ARE BAD: IS IT A MYTH OR SCAM?

We have been bombarded by abundant literature on saturated fats being bad and that they should be avoided in the diet as much as possible. But, the truth of the matter is

THE SATURATED FAT MYTH WASN'T PROVEN IN THE PAST, ISN'T PROVEN TODAY AND NEVER WILL BE PROVEN – BECAUSE IT IS SIMPLY WRONG.

'EATING SATURATED FATS ISN'T BAD FOR YOUR HEALTH. ON THE CONTRARY, IT IS VERY BENEFICIAL.'

Let us see what is meant by saturated fats once again. Chemically, the carbon doesn't have any double bond in their molecule but are linked either to another carbon, hydrogen or oxygen atom. Physically, they are solid at room temperature. This means Ghee and butter are saturated fats. Coconut oil is an exception in a way that most of the fatty acids in coconut oil are saturated, but it is liquid at room temperature.

Now comes the 'most favourite' of us all: unsaturated fats. Mono-unsaturated fats, poly-unsaturated fats etc. Most of the fancy vegetable oils what we see in the market today are unsaturated in variety. They are supposed to confer benefits against coronary artery disease. But, do they really? If so, then how come coronary artery disease cases are on a rise with increased usage of these vegetable oils?

We all know about a blood test known as Serum Lipids. It is the favourite investigation of most physicians nowadays. Physicians use different terms like 'Good Cholesterol' (HDL) and 'Bad Cholesterol' (LDL). Let me simplify them further.

Cholesterol is a variety of fat and fats cannot dissolve in water. Blood is water based; that is it has a water medium with lots of cells, proteins etc. For Cholesterol to be transported in blood, it combines with proteins which make it soluble in water. This chemical which is a combination of fat and proteins is called Lipoprotein which goes by various types known as HDL and LDL. It is said that having high levels of HDL is good for the heart and prevents heart attacks and having high LDL levels makes a person more prone to develop coronary artery disease. But, this is much farther from the truth. Not all LDL is bad. If the size of the LDL particle is large, then it is not associated with coronary heart disease.

Some interesting observations are:-

(1) Saturated fats increase both HDL and the large LDL, which is beneficial in decreasing risk of coronary artery disease.

(2) Serum Cholesterol levels in blood is a flawed marker. It doesn't carry any sense. On the contrary, the latest guidelines published by the American Heart Association say that if your blood Cholesterol levels are high, it indicates that your liver is functioning perfectly.

Some very interesting facts to note here are:-

(1) Since low fat guidelines in the diet are implemented by the 'so called nutrition experts,' obesity has increased.

(2) Since the 'so called cardio-protective vegetable oils' have come in the market, heart disease has increased.

THERE IS NO EVIDENCE TILL DATE THAT SATURATED FATS CAUSE AN INCREASE IN THE RISK OF HAVING HEART ATTACKS. BUT, FOR WHATEVER REASONS, OUR GOVERNMENTS AND HEALTH DEPARTMENTS AND DIETICIANS DON'T WANT TO CHANGE THEIR PERCEPTIONS ABOUT SATURATED FATS.

SOME NUTRITIONAL GUIDELINES TO PREVENT CORONARY ARTERY DISEASE

(1) There should be a correct ratio of Omega 3 and Omega 6 fatty acids in the diet. High quality Omega 3 fatty acids are found in

cold water fish like salmon, sardines, trout, mackerel, eel etc. So, consumption of these fish should increase. The other option is to decrease consumption of Omega 6 fatty acids in the diet. Avoid vegetable and seed oils as well as processed food made from them as they are high in Omega 6 fatty acids.

(2) Trans fats (example is Dalda Ghee) are made by passing hydrogen gas through vegetable oils under high pressure and heat in the presence of a catalyst. Trans fats are responsible for belly fat accumulation, insulin resistance and type II diabetes. They also drastically increase the risk of heart attacks.

Benefits of Coconut Oil

As I said before, we have all been bombarded with false propaganda against saturated fats. And what an absolute lie it is! I am a heart surgeon who has seen thousands of patients in his life. I am a nutritionist and an avid student of the body's biochemistry and I am convinced that saturated fats are amongst our best friends. And I am ready for a debate with any one and prove my point logically. We believe what is told to us by the food industry because they want to sell their products, the pharma companies because they want to sell their costly Cholesterol lowering drugs or the doctors because they believe in the false propaganda and the 'pseudo research' of the pharma companies more than the biochemistry lessons learnt in their first year of medical college.

Coconut oil is the most stable saturated fat in the fat family. Coconut oil burns the slowest, cleanest and sustains a clean fuel source for hours at a time. It is made up of medium chain length fatty acids which are directly used by the body for fuel rather than storing as fat. It stabilises blood sugar levels and do not cause insulin spikes in the blood. It also sustains energy of the body for peak performance. Whenever fatty acids are used as fuel, muscle protein is usually spared.

Other benefits of coconut oil are:

(1) Reduces risk of heart disease.

(2) Cures kidney infection and also, protects the liver.

(3) Lauric acid which is a fatty acid present in coconut oil prevents fungal overgrowth and keeps the internal system clean.

(4) Improves memory.

(5) Improves endurance and boosts energy levels.

(6) Improves all kinds of skin conditions.

(7) Fights and prevents osteoporosis.

Coconut oil is perfect for bodybuilding, fitness and weight loss because it stabilises blood sugar levels and provides a steady source of fuel. It helps in burning off excess body fat.

WHICH COCONUT OIL TO BUY?

Most coconut oils available in the market come from the interior flesh of the coconut known as 'Copra.' Copra is heated to separate the solid interior of the coconut from the oil. Then, the remaining coconut oil is further heated to burn off any moisture and further isolate the oil. These types of coconut oils should be avoided.

Coconut oil that has not been refined or heated or processed is the one to buy. The saturated fats with high levels of MCT (medium chain triglycerides) are present in unrefined coconut oil and this is the right oil to use as it tones the muscle and burns off excess body fat.

So, the take home message is:

Pre-Humans and Humans have been eating saturated fats for thousands of years but, the incidence of heart disease has increased only since 100 years with the advent of vegetable oils.

'BLAMING NEW HEALTH PROBLEMS ON OLD FOODS JUST DOESN'T MAKE SENSE.'

CHAPTER 11

VITAMINS: THE IMPORTANT CO-FACTORS

Vitamins are organic nutrients found in various foods and food supplements. They are required in trace amounts (milligrams or micrograms). Almost all the vitamins cannot be synthesized in the body, hence they are required in the diet. They serve as important co-factors in the chemical reactions taking place in the body i.e. they facilitate and speed up the chemical reactions by taking part in them.

The RDA values for vitamins are not adequate if you are taking vitamins in dosages meant for good health and athletic prowess. RDA values merely indicate the minimum amounts of vitamins that are needed for survival and to prevent deficiency symptoms.

Vitamins are of two kinds:

(1) Those vitamins which are soluble in fat and fat solvents like Vitamin A, D, E and K. They are mostly found in animal foods.

(2) Those Vitamins which are soluble in water. These are the vitamins of the B-complex and Vitamin C.

The fat soluble vitamins

These vitamins can easily dissolve in fat but, not in water, though now some modified water soluble vitamins are synthesized. They are ingested along with the fats in the food and are absorbed in the intestines along with fat. Vitamin D can be synthesized under the skin by the action of ultraviolet rays of sunlight on a compound known as 7-dehydrocholesterol (this is a derivative of cholesterol, another indicator of its usefulness). Some vitamins like vitamin K are also synthesized by the intestinal bacteria, though they are also found in green leafy vegetables. Vitamin A is important for vision, skin, bones and reproduction. Vitamin E acts as a strong antioxidant.

The detailed description of vitamins is beyond the scope of this book. Also, it involves a lots of chemistry, dosages and values, hence I will just broadly outline their functions in the human body and their sources.

VITAMIN A: It is essential for vision, cellular development, fertility and reproduction, integrity of the immune system, healthy skin, hair and the mucous membranes, bone growth, tooth development and immunity against cancer. They are found in liver and fish liver oils, egg yolk, whole milk products and certain crabs. A group of compounds having vitamin A like activity of which Beta Carotene is one form are found in carrots, green leafy vegetables, broccoli, apricots, sweet potato etc. Deficiency can cause symptoms of night blindness, dry skin and mucous membranes and increased infection rate.

VITAMIN D: It is essential for mineralisation of bones by promoting calcium and phosphorus uptake and deposition. It is also important for proper functioning of the nerves and promotion of muscle strength. Deficiency causes soft bones in children leading to a condition known as rickets. In adults, there is an increased tendency for fractures. It is found in abundance in cold water fish and fish liver oils, eggs and whole milk products. It can also be produced under the skin during sunlight exposure.

VITAMIN E: Vitamin E is important for formation of red blood cells in the blood. It is also important in the reproductive process, blood clotting, and cellular division by formation of DNA and RNA and retardation of ageing, cancer formation and heart diseases by its strong anti-oxidant actions. Vitamin E is found in vegetable oils such as sunflower, safflower, soya bean, corn, cotton seed and peanut. Animal sources are usually low in Vitamin E.

VITAMIN K: It mainly takes part in the clotting of blood. Blood clotting is very important otherwise, most of us would die of bleeding from even a minor trauma. Vitamin K is produced chiefly by the bacteria found in your own intestines. Other important source is green leafy vegetables. It is also found in eggs and whole milk products, but in lesser amounts.

Water soluble vitamins

VITAMIN B COMPLEX: This is a group of water soluble vitamins all of them playing important roles in the body.

- ✧ **Thiamine (Vitamin B1)** is necessary for the carbohydrate metabolism i.e. handling and combustion of carbohydrates in your body.

- ✧ **Riboflavin (B2)** is important for energy production and transfer and usage of oxygen at the cellular level.

- ✧ **Niacin (Vitamin B3)** is concerned with energy production of carbohydrates and proteins and also, synthesis of fats and fatty acids in the body.

- ✧ **Pyridoxine (Vitamin B6)** is necessary for breakdown of carbohydrates in the body and formation of amino acids and protein metabolism.

- ✧ **Folate** is essential for multiplication of cells and protein synthesis.

- ✧ **COBALAMINS (Vitamin B12)** is important for multiplication of cells especially nerves and red blood cells in the bone marrow and also energy production. It needs a chemical known as 'intrinsic factor' which is secreted by the digestive juices secreted by the stomach.

- ✧ **Biotin** is an important catalyst for energy production, glucose and fatty acid breakdown, formation of urea resulting from protein breakdown in the body etc. It also enhances fatty acid synthesis and is an important co factor in The Tricarboxylic Acid (TCA) cycle which is the most important chemical pathway in the body for formation of Adenosine Triphosphate (ATP) which is the energy currency of the body. Body uses ATP for all its energy producing activities.

- ✧ **Pantothenic acid** releases energy from carbohydrate and fatty acid breakdown. It is also involved in Cholesterol synthesis and formation of steroid hormones.

- ✧ **Ascorbic Acid (Vitamin C):** It is important in formation of a protein known as collagen which forms the framework of the body's tissues. It is a strong anti-oxidant and protects the tissues against free radical damage. It promotes healthy skin, teeth and gums and also aids in wound healing. It cannot be synthesized by the body and hence, has to be taken in the diet.

Sources of B-Complex Vitamins: Eggs, meat, green leafy vegetables, whole grains, legumes etc. Vitamin C is also found in abundance in citrus fruits like lime, lemons and oranges.

PSEUDOVITAMINS

These are substances similar in their chemical structure to vitamins but, lack the major effects and benefits. They are required by the body in trace amounts daily. Examples are Choline, Para Amino Benzoic Acid, Methionine etc. They have their own functions in the body. Choline for instance, protects against fatty liver. They can be easily available from dietary sources like eggs, meat, liver, green leafy vegetables, whole milk products, legumes etc.

Why fruits in the diet?

We have all been imbibed by the notion that fruits are very essential for health and they contain a lot of vitamins. About the vitamin content, I can say that green leafy vegetables, animal products and whole grains contain much more quantities of vitamins than most fruits with the exception of Vitamin C being present in citrus fruits in good amounts. Moreover, the fruits available in the market are chemically modified nowadays. Apples are wax polished to give them a shining appearance. Chemicals are being injected in fruit to give their pulp a fresh and full look. Chemicals like carbide are used on fruits to give them a lustre. Most of the fruits are stored under cold storage and gradually released in the market. I agree that they provide fibres in your diet, but, more amounts of fibres are found in green leafy vegetables and whole wheat grains. I fail to understand why the virtues of fruits are hyped so much. Of course, fruits are tasty and contain a lot of fructose and glucose which may be used to replenish the body's carbohydrate stores, but then there are cheaper and better sources available for your 'carbohydrate hit.' I am making a very controversial statement in that I believe consuming fruits and fruit juices are more a thing of glamour and 'status symbol' than logical nutrition. Most dieticians and nutritionists might not agree with me but, I am ready to challenge them in a logical debate. After all, this is a book about scientific fitness, not 'broscience.'

CHAPTER 12

MINERALS ARE ALSO IMPORTANT!

Minerals are inorganic substances required by the body. They may be required in large amounts in grams such as sodium, chlorine, potassium and calcium. Some are needed in trace amounts daily such as iron, iodine, manganese, selenium, chromium, boron etc. They are used in various ways in the body. Minerals like sodium, potassium and chlorine maintain the water balance of the body. They also help in transmission of electrical impulses in cells like nerves and muscles. Calcium is responsible for giving hardness to the bones. It also causes muscle contraction. Other minerals are also responsible for various functions in the body as will be explained below.

CALCIUM

It maintains the structure of the bones. It aids in transmission of electrical impulses along the nerves. It forms an important step in the mechanics of muscle contraction. It helps in blood clotting. Good sources are dairy products, cold water fish, broccoli, green leafy vegetables and soft bones.

PHOSPHORUS

It combines with calcium in a chemical bond and gives hardness to the bones. It also forms part of many proteins, lipids and other substances found in the membranes surrounding the cells. ATP and Creatine Phosphate (CrP) which are energy currencies of the body contain phosphate. Sources include most foods containing high amonts of proteins, dairy products and cereals.

THE ELECTROLYTES (SODIUM, POTASSIUM AND CHLORINE)

These are required in comparatively larger quantities daily and are mainly responsible for maintaining the fluid balance in the body, both within and outside the cells. Sodium and chlorine are found in common table salts and most foods. Potassium is found in green leafy vegetables and many fruits. The requirements of electrolytes go up during summer, during heavy exercise where you sweat a lot and dehydration. Sodium is usually absorbed along with glucose so, in times of excess needs, it is always better to drink a glucose solution containing electrolytes, rather than only electrolytes.

MAGNESIUM

It plays a role in muscle and nerve function and heart function. It activates many enzymes which act as catalysts in many chemical reactions. It aids the breakdown of carbohydrates in the body. Sources are whole grains, green leafy vegetables, legumes and certain fruits.

IRON

It forms an important component of haemoglobin which carries oxygen in blood. It is a component of myoglobin found in muscle and also, many enzymes. Sources are red meat, poultry, fish, liver, nuts, legumes, jaggery etc.

ZINC

It contributes to male fertility and is also essential for wound healing. Good sources are meat, liver, nuts, whole grains, fish, oats and dry yeast.

IODINE

It combines with the amino acid tyrosine and forms thyroid hormone within the thyroid gland. Sources are iodized salt, cod, oysters, meat, fish, spinach and dairy products.

SELENIUM

It is a vital component of an enzyme necessary for reversal of oxidative stress known as glutathione peroxidase. It protects against degenerative diseases such as coronary artery disease, arthritis and certain cancers. Sources are nuts, meat, liver, kidney and whole grains.

COPPER

Copper is a part of anti-oxidant enzyme superoxide dismutase which acts as a strong antioxidant and hence, protects against degenerative diseases. It is useful in metabolism and energy production, formation of melanin which is a pigment giving colour to the skin, myelin formation which provides insulation for the nerves and also, increases immunity. Sources include liver, nuts, seafood, cocoa, chocolates, nuts, meat and mushrooms.

MANGANESE

It is required for energy production from carbohydrates, forms collagen which is a protein forming the backbone of all the body's tissues and is a part of the anti-oxidation systems of the body. Sources are meat, green leafy vegetables, whole grains, banana, corn, nuts and cereals.

CHROMIUM

It assists the hormone insulin in bringing down the blood sugar level, increases fatty acid and cholesterol synthesis and also, plays a role in metabolism of DNA and RNA. Good sources are meat, liver, mushrooms, yeast, black pepper, brown rice and potatoes. Insulin cannot work without the presence of Chromium. If any diabetes patient has uncontrolled blood sugars in spite of high insulin dosages, consider chromium deficiency as the cause behind the screen and administer chromium supplementation.

MOLYBDENUM

It helps in production of energy from proteins and also, helps in uric acid production from purines and pyrimidines (DNA and RNA).

FLUORIDE

It leads to strong teeth and increased bone strength. Main source of fluoride in adults is tea. Ground water and nuts also contain fluoride.

BORON

It is required in ultra-small quantities. It is responsible for handling of calcium, phosphorus and magnesium by the body, maintaining intact membranes and also, bone formation. Sources include chickpeas, almonds, beans, vegetables, bananas, walnuts, avocado, broccoli, prunes, oranges, grapes, apples, and legumes.

VANADIUM & GERMANIUM

They are other trace elements which are needed by the body.

CHAPTER 13

ALCOHOL: THE NEMESIS OF MODERN AGE

"It provokes the desire; but, takes away the performance."

– William Shakespeare

The Tragedy of Macbeth, Act II, Scene III.

I come across many clients who give me the impossible task of making them lose weight while they still want to guzzle their way to glory. This chapter will also be of immense benefit to those people who are treading the path of alcohol intake for their de-stressing and entertainment.

Metabolic pathways of alcohol

Alcohol is ingested in form of various drinks like beer, whisky, wine, gin, rum, vodka etc. About 8% of alcohol entering the body gets excreted as such from sweat, urine and breath. Rest of the 92% of alcohol gets metabolised in the body, mainly in the liver. There is an enzyme Alcohol dehydrogenase which breaks down alcohol to acetaldehyde. Acetaldehyde is a poison to the body and is a close relative of formaldehyde (other name is formalin). This acetaldehyde is converted to acetyl radical which combines with another enzyme Coenzyme A. This enters a chain of chemical reactions known as Krebs cycle where it is converted to the energy currency of the body ATP. Alcohol metabolism produces excess amounts of a chemical in the body known as NADH (Nicotinamide Adenine Dinucleotide Hydrogenase) which can lead to lactic acid build up and hypoglycaemia from lack of synthesis of glucose. It can also lead to fat gain and fatty liver.

How alcohol causes fat gain

Alcohol per gram gives 7 kcal. But, it is not only the calories present in alcohol which leads to fat gain. The human body primarily utilises whichever fuel is readily available for its use. Alcohol is rapidly absorbed from the stomach and intestines after ingestion. This is rapidly converted in the liver to the compound acetaldehyde. The breakdown products of acetaldehyde rapidly enters the Krebs cycle which is the main chemical pathway in the body through which ATP is generated. This pathway is used up by the breakdown products of alcohol which makes it a readily available fuel. Till the alcohol is completely metabolised, the utilisation of fats and carbohydrates drops by at least 70%. Moreover, the appetisers like chicken malai tikka, or Paneer tikka (in case of vegetarian drinkers) or chips or fried nuts also add to the calories. Then, after the drinking session, excess food rich in carbohydrates and fats is getting consumed, whose combustion slows down because alcohol provides the ready fuel to the body. Where do you think these calories go to? Obviously, to the fat depots.

Alcohol works differently in different people

- After drinking the same amounts of alcohol, women tend to be more intoxicated than men with a higher blood alcohol level.

- Asians tend to produce more acetaldehyde in their blood after drinking equal amounts of alcohol as Caucasians. 'Flush Syndrome' is very common in Asians. They tend to have increased flushing, sweating, nausea, vomiting and palpitations (awareness of their own heart beat).

- People of older age group tend to become more intoxicated with smaller amounts of alcohol.

- Menopausal females tend to get more intoxicated with smaller amounts of alcohol.

- People with already damaged liver become more intoxicated with smaller amounts of alcohol.

✧ Frequent heavy drinkers become less intoxicated with more and more amounts of alcohol because their enzymes become more efficient in metabolising alcohol. This effect continues till liver failure sets in. After that, their tolerance to alcohol drops rapidly.

Never drink alcohol on an empty stomach

The small intestine is much more efficient in absorbing alcohol than the stomach. If alcohol is drunk on an empty stomach, then, it rapidly enters the intestines where it is quickly absorbed and leads to higher blood alcohol concentration. Presence of food in the stomach slows the emptying of stomach. Fatty foods delays emptying of the stomach by about 3–4 hours. Moreover, drinking alcohol along with meals or after a meal dilutes the alcohol content of the stomach. Hence, it is advisable not to drink on an empty stomach.

How you drink also affects your blood alcohol concentration

✧ Whisky, Rum or Vodka have higher alcohol concentration than beer. Naturally, drinking them will lead to rapid increase in blood alcohol levels as compared to beer.

✧ People drink flavoured drinks more slowly as compared to tasteless drinks. Hence, people who drink neat vodka will tend to drink it faster than drinking whisky.

✧ Carbonated drinks increase the absorption of alcohol.

Short term effects of alcohol

The short term effects of alcohol are the direct result of the quantity of alcohol consumed and also, the rapidity with which it is consumed. Initially, the person feels relaxed, self-confident, and happy and is sociable, but as he/she keeps on drinking, it leads to negative behavioural effects like slurred speech, decreased reflexes, decreased co-ordination, poor judgement and decreased thinking ability, impaired memory and irregular and uncontrolled movements. The person can have violent mood swings, can indulge in unprotected sex and sexual assaults, motor vehicular accidents, suicide, injury and domestic violence. People have also been heard to throw themselves in water and drown.

What is alcoholism?

Drinking alcohol for a long time causes dependency. If a certain quantity causes intoxication in a person, after some time, the same amount may not be enough to cause the same effects. So, the person increases the intake of alcohol. If this drinking continues for a long time, the person drinks more and more quantity to achieve the same effect. Alcoholism leads to long term complications.

LONG TERM COMPLICATIONS OF ALCOHOL

- At some stage, the alcoholic takes only alcohol as his/her main source of calories. There is very poor nutritional intake and hence, nutritional deficiencies develop.
- Liver problems such as fatty liver, alcoholic hepatitis and cirrhosis which develops in the last stage. Cirrhosis is a scarred and shrunken liver. It may cause jaundice, blood in vomit, fluid accumulation and swelling of the legs. Patient may go in deep coma and ultimately it can cause death.
- Stomach ulcers form leading to blood in vomit.
- Diabetes, hypertension, heart attacks and stroke can develop.
- The bones become weak due to loss of calcium and can even fracture when slightly stressed.
- Cancer of breast, food pipe, liver, pancreas, mouth, voice box and throat are linked to alcohol intake.
- The nerves of the body become weak. This can lead to muscle loss and even tingling and numbness.

It is a very common argument amongst drinkers that they always drink under control and hence, they cannot be termed 'alcoholics.' Many self-perpetuated myths are prevalent in the society that alcohol in a little quantity is good for the heart. Let's go over this scenario very carefully. Many of these guys must have started with a small sip and must have progressed up to many pegs without any effects. Quantity definitely increases over time.

And stop equating masculinity with the quantity of alcohol consumed. Alcohol actually decreases the effects of testosterone which is the male hormone and can lead to impotency in the long run.

So, next time you reach out for that glass of whisky, vodka or rum or whatever, remember the words of Shakespeare at the beginning of this narrative. And also keep in mind that you can never transform your body or your mind if you hit the bottle. Give it up.

CHAPTER 14

WATER: THE LEAST DISCUSSED MACRONUTRIENT!

We are all aware of the importance of water in our lives. Water bodies make up almost 70% of the earth's surface. Our bodies are made up of water again up to 65–70%. Different tissues have different water concentrations: blood has more than 80% of its quantity as water, lean muscle has about 70% as water, fat has about 10% of its weight as water, and bones have about 20%. All the chemical reactions of the body take place in water. In spite of knowing this, all of us take this very important macronutrient for granted. Even athletes do not understand the significance of water intake and balance, so what about the general public.

Reduction of even 4% of total body water can hamper your health.

Water balance

The state of hydration of a person is exhibited by his/her water intake and water output.

Water intake occurs by the following routes:

(1) Liquids drunk throughout the day.

(2) Water present in the meals.

(3) Water that is generated in the body as a result of the chemical reactions taking place within.

(4) One gram glucose can hold up to 4 grams of water in the cells.

Water output occurs through the following routes:

(1) **Sweating:** This is the body's natural mechanism for cooling itself. Water gets evaporated from the surface of the skin and this leads

to cooling of the skin. A person can sweat many ounces of water when he/she is exercising in hot climate.

(2) **Urine** is the main route by which water loss happens from the body. The body secretes the products of metabolism through the urine. Many drugs are detoxified and excreted via the urine. During exercise, urinary output drops. Alcohol and coffee increase the urinary output.

(3) **Lungs** is another route by which water loss happens from the body. Water mixes as droplets in the expired air. A person can lose up to 250 ml per day through breathing.

(4) **Faeces** also lead to water loss up to 100 ml per day. In conditions of diarrhoea, there is increased water loss along with loss of electrolytes leading to severe dehydration.

Dehydration and sports performance

Dehydration definitely affects your performance, even if you are a sedentary person or an athlete. As water loss happens from the body, the body's temperature rises, which interferes with many functions of the body. When water loss happens about 4% of the total body weight, the activity efficiency of an individual suffers. Take for instance marathoners and long distance athletes who participate in events during the summer season. They must be losing about a litre of sweat during the race, sometimes more. They have to continuously hydrate themselves during the event otherwise, their performance will suffer. Same goes for non-athletic people too. It has been told to us since childhood that whenever you feel thirsty, you should drink water. But, from a nutritionist's point of view, you should not wait to be thirsty to drink water. By the time you really feel thirsty, the body has already lost a significant amount of water. So, keep drinking water all day long even when you are not thirsty.

How much water to drink?

There is no generalised formula regarding the specific quantity of water that should be consumed. The general rule is that the person should be passing urine at least once every two hours. The colour of the urine should be crystal white. If you are urinating less than that, you should be drinking more water. You should not be waiting for yourself to feel thirsty to drink water. You should be hydrating yourself continuously. Try for at least 6–7 litres of water per day. Then, see your skin glowing.

What about rehydration drinks?

Along with water, the body also excretes a lot of electrolytes. This loss can be from sweat, urine or faeces. It is necessary to take electrolytes along with water for rehydration. The main electrolytes are sodium and chlorine which maintain the water balance of the body. Sodium is absorbed along with glucose. Hence, the ideal rehydrating drink should have glucose as one of its ingredients. But, for non-athletic people, simple water is preferable to fruit juices and the carbonated beverages as they lead to unnecessary calorie intake.

CHAPTER 15

OXYGEN: THE ELIXIR OF LIFE

We all know that oxygen is necessary for life. Without oxygen, life is not possible on this earth. The air that we breathe in contains 20% oxygen. During inspiration, the lungs expand and take in the air. The oxygen in the inhaled air diffuses through the walls of the small air sacs called alveoli. This oxygen is taken up by the small blood vessels called capillaries. It combines with the pigment Haemoglobin present in the red blood cells in the blood. This oxygen gets transported via blood to the tissues where haemoglobin releases oxygen which is used by the cells for their function and damage repair.

Now, just imagine that your body has more oxygen to use. Wouldn't that be nice! Can it be achieved? Oxygen is not like a cold drink which you can drink as much as you need. There are specific ways to increase its availability and utilisation. Don't believe me? Keep on reading.

The lungs expand in a passive way. There is negative pressure between the lungs and the rib cage. That means that there is vacuum. The lungs do not expand by themselves. The muscles of the chest wall expand the rib cage, so that there is an increase in volume inside the chest. Since there is already vacuum between the lungs and the chest wall, the lungs expand passively. Air is sucked into the lungs as a result of this vacuum.

With this basic picture in mind, let me show you how oxygen delivery and utilisation can be increased in the body.

- By a proper combination of weight training and cardio, the muscles around the chest wall and upper back can be developed. These muscles by their contraction, expand the chest wall vigorously thus, enhancing the capacity of the lungs to suck in more air. More air means more oxygen, right!

✧ By a judicious plan of cardio, the quality of the lung tissue can be significantly improved. The capacity of the lung tissue to take in more air and better oxygen transfer increases.

✧ Intense weight training combined with correct form of cardio leads to thickening of the heart muscle with increased force of contraction. The heart rate also comes down as the pumping of the heart increases.

✧ The blood vessels supplying the tissues become better in quality by exercise. They increase in size and number and hence, can accommodate more blood. This leads to better oxygen delivery to the tissues.

✧ Exercise can increase the blood volume by more than a litre. Proper nutrition can increase the haemoglobin in the blood cells. This increases oxygen delivery to the body's tissues.

So, the summary is that correct exercises combined with correct nutrition can make your body use more oxygen than it normally does. Your work efficiency will increase and you will feel energetic throughout the day.

CHAPTER 16

THE DARK SIDE OF OXYGEN: TOXIC FREE RADICALS

In the previous chapter, oxygen is described as an elixir of life. It is absolutely essential for life and life cannot exist without the presence of oxygen, at least not on the planet earth. We saw various techniques by which oxygen delivery to the tissues can be increased. But, do you know that oxygen has a dark side too and is responsible for the ageing process and also, various diseases especially those occurring at an older age like arthritis, diabetes, coronary artery disease and even certain cancers? Strange, but true!

What are free radicals?

To understand what free radicals are, I need to give you a very brief refresher course in physical chemistry. The human body is composed of many types of cells. These cells are made up of many different types of molecules. The molecules are made up of atoms of different elements. Now, if you remember from your school days, the atoms are composed of a nucleus in the centre which contains neutrons and protons. Protons are positively charged energy particles and neutrons do not have any charge. This positive charge of the centre of the atom is exactly balanced by the same number of negatively charged energy particles rotating around the centre. These negative particles are known as electrons.

Now, the atoms form bonds by combining with other atoms. Atoms try to fill their outer orbits with electrons from other atoms. The electrons which are present in the outer orbit are shared by these atoms which are joining together. As a result, the atoms try to reach a steady and stable state.

Normally, these bonds are so stable that they do not break. But, sometimes, weak bonds split in a way that one of the atoms is left with an unpaired electron. Hence, it becomes unstable. This is called a free radical. These free radicals attack the nearest stable molecule and try to share its electron so that it becomes stable. But, this leaves the other molecule with an unpaired electron and hence, it becomes unstable in turn and attacks its nearest molecule and makes it unstable. This causes a chain reaction which ultimately leads to death of a living cell.

Free radicals are normally formed in the body. The body's immune system creates free radicals to fight against bacteria and viruses.

Free radicals are also formed due to environmental factors such as pollution, radiation, cigarette smoking and many herbicides and pesticides. Even intense exercise especially endurance activities like marathons, long distance cycling, triathlons and similar others generate a lot of free radicals.

Normally, the body can handle these free radicals. But, if free radicals become excessive, then damage to the cells and tissues can occur. Free radical damage accumulates with age and is the primary reason for ageing.

Diseases thought to be caused by free radical damage

- ✧ Multi organ diseases like ageing, chronic fatigue and diabetes.
- ✧ Eyes: Cataracts, macular and retinal degeneration.
- ✧ Blood vessels: Atherosclerosis, narrowing of the arteries, damage to the inner lining of arteries and veins, hypertension.
- ✧ Heart: Coronary artery disease, Cardiac fibrosis, hypertension, heart attacks.
- ✧ Skin: Sunburn, ageing and wrinkles, psoriasis, dermatitis, cancer of the skin known as melanoma.
- ✧ Kidney: Chronic renal disease, Nephritis.
- ✧ Joints: Rheumatoid arthritis, Osteoarthritis.
- ✧ Lung: Chronic lung problems, Asthma, allergies, cancer.

- ✧ Brain: Alzheimer's disease, Parkinsonism, migraine, stroke, cancer.
- ✧ Immune system: Auto-immune diseases, Lupus, Irritable bowel syndrome, multiple sclerosis, cancers.

How anti-oxidants may prevent against free radical damage and prevent degenerative diseases

Anti-oxidants neutralise free radicals by donating one of their own electrons, thus ending the 'electron stealing reactions' of the free radicals. The antioxidants themselves do not become free radicals because they are stable in either form. They act as scavengers of free radicals, helping to prevent cell and tissue damage that could lead to degenerative diseases.

Toxic free radicals and their role in lipid peroxidation

We are what we eat. If you take more of saturated fats, your body and cell membranes will primarily be composed of saturated fats. On the other hand, if your diet consists predominantly of unsaturated fats, then your body fat contains more of unsaturated fats.

Polyunsaturated fats contain double bonds between carbon atoms. These bonds are slightly more unstable than the chemical structure of saturated fat. These double bonds tend to get affected more by oxygen free radicals and undergo a chemical process known as lipid peroxidation. This chemical reaction causes more damage to the cell. Hence, if the polyunsaturated fats in your body increase beyond a certain limit, then, this fat is more prone to damage by these oxygen free radicals. Maybe, that is the reason why food cooked in saturated fats lasts longer than that cooked in polyunsaturated fats. This may be considered as another argument in favour of saturated fats.

CHAPTER 17

ANTI-OXIDANTS AND THEIR ROLE IN PREVENTION OF DEGENERATIVE DISEASES

In the previous chapter, we saw how everything in excess is harmful. What takes birth has to end. Nature has its roots of destruction built within its own infrastructure. During times of stress as mentioned previously, the very same oxygen which gives us life can form highly toxic radicals which can oxidise the body's own tissues and damages them. This is the very reason why living things age, degenerate and die. If this process is left unchecked, death would come swiftly to us. Fortunately, there are certain in-built mechanisms in the body which provide a defence mechanism against these toxic free radicals. This slows down the cellular damage and its resulting degeneration and death. Previously, it was thought that these anti-oxidants had no role in reducing the oxidative stress of the body, but, now strong evidence is coming to light which suggests their efficacy in prolonging life by at least 5–8 years.

Anti-oxidants are by nature stable compounds. They exchange electrons with these free radicals, thus reducing their number. One question may arise that is how these anti-oxidants are able to stabilise themselves? It so happens that even if they exchange electrons with these radicals, they remain in a stable state both ways. Some of these anti-oxidants may transfer their electrons through some chemical pathways in the body and thus, neutralise these free radicals.

The inbuilt mechanisms of the human body against free radical damage are:

- ✧ **Uric acid** is by far the most important anti-oxidising agent in the human body. It has the highest anti-oxidant property in the blood, almost 50%. It reacts against oxidants like peroxynitrite, peroxides and hypochlorous acid. As the uric acid concentration increases in the blood, so does its anti-oxidant properties. It has especially strong anti-oxidant properties at high altitudes. This is disproportionate to the risk of gout that it entails.

- **Glutathione** is a protein found in animals and is synthesized in the cells. It has very strong anti-oxidant properties.

- **Melatonin** is a powerful anti-oxidant. It easily crosses cell membranes and also, acts on the brain.

- **Vitamin C** (Ascorbic acid) is an oxidation-reduction catalyst found in plants and animals. Humans cannot synthesize Vitamin C in their bodies, hence it must be taken in the diet.

- **Vitamin E** is a collective name for eight chemicals called Tocopherols and Tocotrienols. They are fat soluble vitamins. They protect cell membranes from oxidation by reacting with lipid radicals formed in the lipid peroxidation reactions.

- **Beta Carotene** is also a strong anti-oxidant.

Different anti-oxidants are said to benefit different body parts

- **Beta-Carotene** is said to promote eye health.

- **Lycopene** enhances prostate health.

- **Flavonoids** preserve the heart muscle.

- **Proanthocyanidins** promote the health of urinary tract.

- **Astaxanthin and Vitamin E** is good for skin. Here, I would like to add that limiting sunlight exposure and using a strong sunscreen throughout life protects more against sunlight induced oxidative damage. Topical Vitamin A, C and E are also said to prevent skin damage by ultraviolet light induced free radicals, but using a sunscreen with SPF 30 would give more benefit.

✧ **Astaxanthin and Spirulina** confer benefit by boosting the immunity by reducing free radical damage to the immune system acquired during its fight with bacteria and viruses.

Can anti-oxidants do more harm than good?

It has been postulated that some anti-oxidants may do more harm than good in humans under certain conditions. Hypothetically, free radicals may induce an endogenous response (body's response) that may protect against free radicals from outside the body and possibly other toxic compounds that are either formed in the body or introduced from outside. It is suggested that free radicals may increase life span and this increase may be offset by anti-oxidants. But, now more and more evidence is accumulating in favour of anti-oxidants as a preventive measure in cases of degenerative diseases mentioned in the previous chapter.

CHAPTER 18

ERGOGENIC AIDS

Ergogenic aids are the various different means by which performance and health are said to be enhanced.

They can be classified as:-

(1) Nutritional ergogenic supplements.

(2) Mechanical ergogenic aids.

(3) Psychological ergogenic aids.

NUTRITIONAL ERGOGENIC SUPPLEMENTS

They are dietary supplements that supposedly enhance performance and health. They are taken routinely by athletes to gain that competitive edge. Nowadays, many athletic competitions are won by 1/100th of a second, hence it is the wish of every athlete to have that extra advantage over others.

By definition, a supplement is something which is taken other than the diet to meet the nutritional needs. But, athletes take them to enhance their performance. This type of supplementation has been in place since a long time. Previously, hunters used to kill and eat the heart of lions and deer because they felt that these practices will gain them extra courage, boldness, swiftness and killer instinct.

Dietary supplements are a billion dollar industry. The industry targets the entire population range from a sedentary individual to elite athletes. These manufacturing companies do not have to prove that these supplements are safe and that they work. As a result, they make such blanket statements and get away with disclaimers like "This product has not been evaluated by the FDA (Food and Drug Administration).

It is not intended to diagnose, prevent or treat disease." Most of these products do not have any scientific evidence which says that they are effective. Often the studies that are quoted to show their efficacy are never found in other scientific journals. Even if the studies are authentic, they are never performed on the sample of the population that are actually going to use the product.

Manufacturers use the word "natural" for their supplements. Many people and athletes fall for these 'natural' supplements thinking that natural means 'safe' and 'legal.' But, that is not so all the time. Many ephedrine-containing substances might be natural but, they are by no means safe and legal.

Governing organizations such as Natural Collegiate Athletic Association (NCAA) and International Olympic Committee (IOC) have published lists of banned substances which will disqualify the athlete from competing if the athlete tests positive for one of these banned substances. The NCAA says that not knowing whether a substance is on the banned list is not an acceptable excuse for a positive drug test.

Newer supplements are hitting the market almost daily with tall claims of stunning transformations and superhuman performances. Many elite athletes are asked to endorse these products by proclaiming that they have been using them since ages and they are the reason for their trophies and awards. To determine whether a supplement is safe and effective, I suggest you research thoroughly before emptying your wallet. You should exercise caution when the following statements appear as regarding a product:

- ✧ Boasts that it is quick and easy.
- ✧ Uses testimonials from 'real users' such as elite athletes and professional bodybuilders.
- ✧ Gives a generalised statement that it is applicable for each and every one.
- ✧ Goes against scientific and medical evidence.
- ✧ Claims that it has been in use since ancient times.

✧ The product has a secret formulation known only to the manufacturer.

ANDROSTENEDIONE

Androstenedione is formed in the body during the synthesis of testosterone. Despite claims that it increases muscle mass, it has not been proven to be as efficacious as it claims. It is not recommended in pregnant women, adolescents and people with medical diseases like coronary artery disease, hypertension or prostate enlargement.

DEHYDROEPIANDROSTERONE (DHEA)

DHEA is a hormone mainly produced in your adrenal glands. It is also formed in the testis in the testosterone producing pathway. Medically, DHEA is not recommended below the age of forty years in males because their bodies are already making enough DHEA and there is no use to give it in supplementation. Its beneficial effects have not yet been proved but it seems to confer some physical and psychological benefit to male athletes over the age of forty years and in female athletes. It is banned by most sports committees and hence, should not be used.

BRANCHED CHAIN AMINO ACIDS

BCAAs are marketed as preserving muscle during exercise, increase exercise endurance and prevent fatigue. There is a big hype in the market regarding their efficacy and use. But, clinical research has not conclusively proved the effectiveness of BCAAs in increasing exercise performance or endurance. Sufficient quantities of BCAAs are obtained from high protein diets. Hence, there is no evidence to indicate that athletes need extra supplementation. Ingestion of carbohydrate drinks during workouts have a better role.

CAFFEINE

Caffeine has been claimed to increase energy, increase fat loss and increase endurance. It acts as a stimulant of the brain and decreases fatigue. It is also said to increase force of muscle contraction and facilitates fat utilisation. Taking caffeine pre-workout can increase its intensity. But, make sure that your sport allows you to take caffeine as it is banned in certain sports.

CHROMIUM PICOLINATE

Chromium is a co-factor to insulin action. It potentiates the action of insulin by sensitizing body's tissues to insulin. It increases protein synthesis by increasing the uptake and utilisation of amino acids. Chromium is widely obtained from various dietary sources and usually doesn't need extra supplementation.

CREATINE

Creatine is known to increase power output of the muscles during high intensity exercise and activity. This is amply proved in many research studies. It increases total body weight especially fat free mass.

CONJUGATED LINOLEIC ACID (CLA)

CLA has been claimed to increase lean body mass and decrease fat percentage. They are naturally occurring fatty acids found in meat and dairy products. It is claimed to increase hormonal responses in cells thereby leading to anabolism (growth). But, there is no conclusive evidence to prove these claims.

GLUCOSAMINE

Glucosamine is a sugar formed from glucose and amino acids and plays an important role in forming the structure of cartilage, tendons and ligaments. In theory, glucosamine should repair damaged cartilages, but actual evidence suggests that it plays a role in regeneration of cartilage in the early stages of Osteoarthritis. During later stages, glucosamine role is yet to be proved.

L-CARNITINE

L-Carnitine is an amine made by the body. Its main role is that it transports fatty acids for oxidation and energy production in structures known as mitochondria which generate power within cells. Mitochondria are power producing factories within cells which generate ATP from carbohydrates, proteins and fats. This action might be considered important in that L-Carnitine might increase the fat burning process. But, clinical research studies have not conclusively proved its role in fat loss.

COENZYME Q10 (UBIQUINONE)

Coenzyme Q10 is an enzyme found in every mitochondria. It participates in the production of ATP from glucose and fatty acids. It is supposed to provide energy for long distance events such as marathons by continuously oxidising the fuels available to the cell for constant energy. Clinical studies in athletes give equivocal results.

GAMMA ORYZANOL AND FERRULIC ACID

These supplements are thought to have a variety of metabolic effects such as endorphin release, anti-oxidation, stress reduction, growth and recovery. But, clinical results are sparse.

GLYCEROL

Glycerol is a molecule which forms the backbone of fat in the body. It is a three-carbon molecule and attached to three fatty acids. When fat becomes mobilised from fat stores and is split by enzymes, it results in formation of three fatty acids and one molecule of glycerol. This glycerol is used as emollient (smoothening agent) in skin care products and cosmetics and also as a sweetening agent in medicine syrups. Glycerol is a constituent in certain hydration fluids used during long distance sports to maintain proper hydration in athletes.

INOSINE

Inosine forms a part of ATP (Adenosine Triphosphate) which is the energy currency of the body. It is shown to increase energy during strenuous workouts and also endurance sports.

BIOFLAVONOIDS

Bioflavonoids are the brightly coloured chemical compounds found in fresh fruits and vegetables. They are supposed to assist Vitamin C in its absorption and action. They are supposed to have strong anti-oxidant properties. The ergogenic effects of bioflavonoids have not yet been proved, but they are supposed to enhance recovery after strenuous exercise and reduce stress.

BETA-HYDROXY BETA-METHYLBUTYRATE (BHMB)

BHMB is one of the newer metabolites to enter the weightlifting and bodybuilding market. It is said to promote nitrogen retention, which means more amino acids are available for protein synthesis. It is now being brandished as a molecule for muscle gain. Remember, that BHMB has to be used as a supplement along with strict exercise and nutrition program in bodybuilding and not singly.

ALKALINIZERS AND BLOOD BUFFERS

Sodium bicarbonate is now being touted as a blood buffer. It is claimed that it reduces muscle cramps and combats the acidity built up in the blood as a result of lactic acidosis resulting from very prolonged and strenuous exercise. Studies performed on sprinters and medium distance runners have proved its value. It is also used as an antacid. Use of Sodium Bicarbonate may lead to bloating and flatulence. Use with caution in hypertension.

MELATONIN

Melatonin is a sleep producing substance formed in the body. It has not been proven to benefit health or to improve athleticism. Nevertheless, it has been postulated to induce a sound and longer lasting sleep thus, enhancing recovery. But, nothing is proved so far.

GINSENG

There are three types of Ginseng used for many centuries. It has been claimed to increase energy levels and reduce stress. The three types are Chinese Ginseng, Siberian Ginseng and American Ginseng. Formulations containing 2–4% Ginseng are available in the market. The various research studies performed for the effect of Ginseng have produced conflicting results. Ginseng is a component of good multi-vitamins/minerals supplements.

HERBS

Herbs have long been used by humans for health. Some herbs form part of a healthy diet and some form ingredients for various herbal medicines or potions. These herbs can be of use to an athlete or an exercising individual. But, their use has to be done under strict guidance of a herbologist or a person who has a thorough knowledge of herbs. Your doctor will definitely not know anything about herbs. Herbs used correctly may give you an extra edge over other individuals, but, if used in a wrong way, they can have disastrous results as well. There is an Asian herbal practice of using herbs to balance the flow of energy. Another practice is to use herbs for their specific actions e.g. Caffeine content in guarana. Both approaches are sound. If you seek to be a professional athlete, then you should definitely use herbs in your supplementation. Herbs come in many forms: whole herbs to make tea with or as tablets or soft gels or as potions and herbal extracts. Standardized herbal products are what you should aim for as many herbal products also have side-effects if taken in too large a dose.

MECHANICAL ERGOGENIC AIDS

Mechanical forms of ergogenic aids include specially designed clothing, enhanced forms of sports equipment and/or some physical devices in contact with a person's body.

Some examples of mechanical ergogenic aids are:

- ✧ Altitude training.
- ✧ Heart rate monitors.
- ✧ Computers used for analysis of various parameters like VO2 max etc.

- ✧ Video recorders to analyse technique.
- ✧ Weights.
- ✧ Parachutes.
- ✧ Elastic cords (resistance tubing).
- ✧ Uphill and downhill running.
- ✧ Weighted vests.
- ✧ Sports clothing, footwear and other equipment.
- ✧ Timing equipment.

All of these mechanical aids are just used to enhance the training of an athlete and are perfectly legal.

PSYCHOLOGICAL ERGOGENIC AIDS

These techniques are easy to learn and can be practised anywhere:

- ✧ Hypnosis to distract the mind from negative thoughts before an event.
- ✧ Cheering.
- ✧ Positive visualisation.
- ✧ Soothing music.
- ✧ Deep breathing techniques and relaxation.
- ✧ Yoga can relax tension in the muscles and the mind.

These are various performance enhancing aids for maintaining good health in an individual and also increase performance of an athlete. As regarding the nutritional ergogenic aids, please research and then only try them out. My advice to the athletes is that these nutritional and mechanical ergogenic aids are costly and not easily available. Tall claims have been made regarding the nutritional supplements but, research is showing conflicting results in most cases. So, the ball is in your court now.

USE OF PERFORMANCE ENHANCING DRUGS IN ATHLETES AND BODYBUILDING

The main idea behind this book is to promote fitness and bodybuilding naturally. But, let me put in a word here that these compounds are used extensively by bodybuilders as they promote growth of lean body mass, much beyond the physiological range. During the leaning phase, when the physique athletes are on hypocaloric diets, these compounds are used to preserve lean body mass. Abuse of these substances are harmful to the body. They can be the cause of liver or kidney failure. All the sports, except professional bodybuilding have banned the use of these substances. Very few bodybuilders openly admit that they have taken steroids and peptides as part of their pre-competition preparations.

The aping of these athletes is so prevalent now that youngsters are resorting to these substances for getting a lean and ripped look of their heroes. Bodybuilding competitions are very common nowadays and hence, more and more young athletes, including females are hooked onto these drugs. These drugs play havoc with your sex hormones and their associated metabolic effects. Even if you aspire to become a physique model or a professional bodybuilder, that does not give you an excuse to inject yourself indiscriminately. Safe prescription of these drugs under the guidance of a super-specialist who has exquisite knowledge of this 'dark side of bodybuilding' is still tolerable. But, please do not listen to uncertified people who only have their financial interests at heart.

CHAPTER 19

THE GLUTEN HOAX

Gluten is the latest nutrient to get the 'stick' in the fitness industry. If you walk down a supermarket selling food items or go through a restaurant menu, it is becoming very common to see the words 'Gluten free' leaping out at you. Many people jump on the band-wagon and follow a gluten-free diet and go for fruits and vegetables as part of healthy living. Others avoid gluten because they consider themselves 'gluten-intolerant.' Some even imagine themselves as having a milder form of Coeliac disease (this is a disorder in which consumption of gluten causes damage to the small intestine).

Whether eating a gluten-free diet is a matter of choice or necessity to you, I think you should know everything about this latest fad.

So, what exactly is Gluten?

Gluten is not a man-made toxic chemical that is added to the food. It is a natural protein found in wheat, barley and rye. It gives form and texture to pastas and breads. Along with yeast, it is responsible for swelling of the bread during baking.

Nowadays, the latest fad in the fitness industry is to go for gluten-free diets. The fitness industry is trying to propagate that all the world's population might be gluten-intolerant and hence, should avoid gluten in their diet. And, we Indians are always the first to jump on the band wagon. Sheer idiocy! Indians have been eating chapattis and parathas since centuries and suddenly, we find ourselves to be gluten-intolerant just because some 'fitness expert' said so. Less than 0.1% of the Indian population is gluten sensitive. And, Coeliac disease is extremely rare in India. If you remove gluten from your diet, your body is likely to receive lesser amounts of Vitamin B Complex, Iron and Dietary fibre. Scientific research indicates that eating whole grains containing gluten can lower the risk of diabetes mellitus type II and Cardio-Vascular disease. So, unless you are diagnosed as gluten-intolerant (that is the domain of a gastroenterologist, not your gym trainer), it is perfectly 'safe' to eat wheat and still remain healthy.

Gluten and fitness

My one question to all the 'self-styled fitness gurus is: "Please logically, scientifically and medically explain how gluten stands in the way of achieving a dream physique?"

The fitness world has equated gluten-free diets to fat loss. There is no evidence, I repeat NO EVIDENCE to support the statement that when calories and macronutrients are controlled, foods containing gluten will not result in fat loss.

Just like any other fad diet, if a person avoids gluten and eats only fruits and vegetables as part of his/her carbohydrate fulfilment, then the drop in the overall calories will lead to fat loss, not avoidance of gluten.

Diagnosing Gluten sensitivity

Many fitness freaks believe that following a gluten-free diet leads to improved exercise performance. This will be true only when you are gluten sensitive. People make 'self-diagnosis' of gluten sensitivity when they feel bloating and flatulence after eating wheat products. But, this bloating can also be due to the oil, spices or certain vegetables present in their meals. Coeliac disease is diagnosed only after many blood investigations and intestinal biopsies. So, if you are experiencing digestive issues, your first step should be to evaluate and reassess your overall dietary patterns. Sometimes, a simple remedy such as digestive enzymes can control most of these symptoms, rather than cutting out wheat altogether from your diet.

Should we go gluten free?

I am a doctor and a nutritionist. I find very little evidence to state that if wheat is removed from the diet, health and performance are improved.

But, removing wheat will definitely lessen your intake of other nutrients like Vitamins and Iron. If you still feel that you have the symptoms of gluten sensitivity, it is better to consult a Gastroenterologist for eliminating or confirming the diagnosis.

Think logical! Act scientific! Be SCIENTIFIT!

CHAPTER 20

BRANCHED CHAIN AMINO ACIDS (BCAA)

BCAA is a collective name for a group of three amino acids which have side branches in their molecules as part of their chemical structure. Simply speaking, the three amino acids are Leucine, Isoleucine and Valine, out of which Leucine seems to be the most important. They make up about 35% of the amino acids which make up your muscle proteins and almost 40% of the amino acids in the diet. Meat, dairy products and legumes are rich sources of BCAA. BCAA can be absorbed in a single form from the gut and they directly go to the blood circulation. They are essential amino acids meaning, they cannot be synthesized in the body and have to be taken in the diet. They are much touted in the bodybuilding world as one of the most essential supplements for muscle building and especially for preserving muscle in the 'cutting stage' when the athletes go for the super lean look.

How BCAA are important for the body?

✧ BCAA promote protein synthesis via signalling the chemical pathways in the body's cells especially muscle. Leucine seems to be especially important in this regard. The BCAA are part of whey protein, but, they are chemically bound to other amino acids in whey and hence, their digestion and absorption takes a few hours. But, if taken as amino acid preparation in a single form, they are rapidly absorbed into the blood stream and hit the target tissue especially muscle. Leucine also initiates insulin secretion from the pancreas. This hormone insulin drives the amino acids into the cells. Leucine also initiates several chemicals inside the cells especially muscle and hence, muscle protein synthesis occurs and the muscle grows.

- During the fat loss phase in normal people as well as athletes and bodybuilders when the subjects are on a calorie deficit diet, the body tries hard to hold on to the fat stores and burn up the muscle as some of the amino acids are glucogenic that is they can be converted to glucose by the body and used as fuel. Also, some amino acids can be directly oxidised as fuel. If these people are supplemented with extra BCAA, they can preserve a lot of their muscle during the calorie deficit phase.

- When muscle hypertrophy (growth) occurs in athletes and also in exercising individuals, the muscle burns its own Leucine stores even at rest. Hence, these subjects need to be supplemented with BCAA, especially Leucine. Now, BCAA are commonly found in protein rich diets. Hence, this characteristic of the muscle can be offset even without BCAA intake at regular intervals.

- BCAA decreases fatigue during exercise and provides energy. During exercise, there is a gradual increase of a chemical known as Serotonin (5-HT) in the brain. The raw material for 5-HT is an amino acid known as Tryptophan. This tryptophan is found circulating in the blood in a free state and also as a combination with the blood protein albumin. Tryptophan enters the brain via blood and leads to increased production of 5-HT in the brain which causes fatigue and drowsiness during exercise. If a person is exercising in a fasted state, then he/she utilises a large amount of fat as fuel. Free fatty acids are circulating in the blood. They displace tryptophan from its protein combination and increase free tryptophan in the blood which crosses over to the brain. BCAA, if supplemented before and during exercise, leads to its oxidation for energy, thus decreasing the mobilisation of fatty acids from the fat stores, thereby indirectly decreasing the amount of free tryptophan in the blood. This invigorating effect of BCAA during exercise is weaker as compared to the ingestion of a carbohydrate drink during exercise as this glucose will act as the fuel and will decrease fat mobilisation. Glucose will also provide the brain with adequate energy and hence, will prevent fatigue.

Formulations available and dosage of BCAA

BCAA are available in various formulations as tablets, powders or liquids. The Leucine content of these formulations is double that of Isoleucine and Valine as it is the main BCAA that is actively at work in the body, though the other two are no less important. BCAA have also been combined with other amino acids like glutamine, arginine and citrulline maleate.

The exact dosage of BCAA is difficult to calculate but, can range from 5–20 grams per dose taken at intervals during the day.

Is it a 'MUST' to take BCAA?

BCAA are commonly present in high protein diets in adequate amounts. Rich food sources are meat, dairy products and legumes. Researches have indicated that if your diet contains a high protein intake up to 2 grams/kg of body weight, then you needn't take BCAA. So, for a common man who is looking to build muscle as part of remaining fit and if the person is a non-vegetarian, then BCAA probably has no role. Same is the case with most athletes who are fed high protein diets. For bodybuilders, since their physique is more important than any athletic performance and they need to be super lean and dry when they step on stage, they have a strong contention for BCAA supplementation. But, for the general public, I still feel dietary manipulation will suffice.

CHAPTER 21

ANATOMY OF THE HUMAN BODY: CELLS, TISSUES AND SYSTEMS

The human body is a complex assembly of various systems which even though separate, are interdependent upon each other to sustain life. There are various systems in the human body namely skeletal system, muscular system, nervous system, cardio-vascular system, endocrine system, respiratory system, urinary system, reproductive system etc. If you observe carefully, their functions and workings might be different, but each system needs the help of other systems to function optimally. Each of these systems are made up of various tissues and each of these tissues are made up of cells which are the smallest units of life.

What is a cell?

The cell is the smallest and the most fundamental unit of life. Just as every molecule has atoms as their building blocks, so are cells as they form the building blocks of every tissue. There are more than 100 trillion cells in the human body. Even though cells may differ in structure and function, but still they possess the same genetic material. Somehow, these 100 trillion cells arrange and organise themselves into forming a complex phenomenon called 'The human body.' The primary quality of the cells which define them as a living tissue is that most cells can divide themselves. The human body initially starts as an egg cell which comes from the mother and a sperm cell which comes from the father. The union of these two cells (we call them gametes) forms a cell called as a 'Zygote.' This zygote divides and re-divides itself and then, gets embedded into the wall of the uterus which is also called the female reproductive sac. The cell division continues here and then, the cells start differentiating themselves into cells of various tissues like nervous tissue, muscle, connective tissue, bones, reproductive tissue etc. These tissue cells then further rearrange themselves to form the ultimate phenomenon called 'The human body.'

We say that cells are the fundamental units of life. Each cell has the ability to survive independently. If you magnify the cell under a microscope, you will see that the cell is a complex structure in itself vibrating with life. There are various sub-structures in the cells known as 'Organelles.' Let us look at these components of the cell individually as this knowledge will be very important in our goal that is 'SCIENTIFIC AND LOGICAL FITNESS.'

CELL MEMBRANE

If there is a structure called cell, then it has to have a boundary wall. This boundary wall is a layer formed by lipids (fats) and proteins and is called the cell membrane or Plasma membrane. This membrane contains the cell. It also allows transfer of nutrients to and from the interior of the cell to outside the cell. This transfer can be 'passive' i.e. not requiring energy for the transfer or 'active' i.e. requiring energy. This membrane also contains molecules called 'receptors' which bind with certain chemicals coming from other organs like hormones which act as 'signals' so that certain chemical reactions can take place within the cells.

The cell membranes of certain cells like nerves can also pass electric current along its length by a complex play of electrolytes.

CYTOPLASM

The cell is a bag of liquid contained within its cell membrane. This liquid is known as cytoplasm. Cytoplasm contains the nucleus and various organelles of the cell. This is the place where various chemical reactions take place such as breaking down of glucose molecule (glycolysis).

NUCLEUS

Nucleus is the command centre of the cell. It usually lies in the centre of the cell and contains the genetic material DNA which is in the form of structures known as 'Chromosomes.' All of us know that the entire genetic material is coded on the DNA. The signals for formation of various molecules is given by the DNA in the form of a chemical known as RNA which passes out of the nucleus into the cytoplasm where it forms proteins and other molecules. Nucleus also helps in cell division. The chromosomes have the capacity to replicate themselves and that's how nuclear division takes place followed by the cell division and growth of the tissue and individual.

MITOCHONDRIA

Mitochondria are the chemical factories of the cell. The energy currency of the body ATP is formed in the mitochondria. Various molecules like glucose and fatty acids are broken down here. Whenever the chemical bond between atoms break, energy is released. This energy is trapped in the mitochondria in the form of ATP. Molecules like l-carnitine increase the transfer of fatty acids inside the mitochondria. That's why this supplement is being touted as a fat loss supplement, though how much it aids in fat loss is still to be decided upon. There is a chain of chemical reactions known as 'Krebs cycle' which takes place in the mitochondria in presence of oxygen. The ATP is released from the mitochondria during muscle contractions and other chemical reactions which require energy.

RIBOSOMES

These are small spherical organelles which play a very important role in protein synthesis.

ENDOPLASMIC RETICULUM

They are a network of canals in the cytoplasm. They act as transport roadways of various molecules within the cell as well as molecular transport outside the cell. They are of two types, rough and smooth. Rough endoplasmic reticulum has ribosomes attached to them, hence proteins can be synthesized there and transported anywhere within the cell or outside the cell. Smooth endoplasmic reticulum does not contain ribosomes. Its function is not known, though it is speculated that smooth endoplasmic reticulum is involved in cholesterol metabolism and steroid hormone synthesis.

GOLGI APPARATUS

Golgi apparatus or Golgi bodies are spherical sac like structures in the cell and are believed to be the site of synthesis of glycogen molecules. They are also involved in transport of these molecules outside the cell.

LYSOSOMES

Lysosomes are sac like structures found within the cell. They contain digestive enzymes which serve as catalysts and can break down any component of the cell that is any type of protein, carbohydrate and fat. Lysosomes swell in size when they are active. The breakdown products can be used for re-synthesis of other molecules or can be expelled as waste products from the cell. Lysosomes serve to destroy the bacteria trapped within the White Blood Cells. These lysosomes are also called 'suicidal bags' because they can release their enzymes and cause cell death.

Tissues

Groups of cells form various tissues. Tissues in varied form and proportion form organs. Different organs form a system.

Types of tissues are:

(1) Epithelial tissues.

(2) Connective tissues.

(3) Muscle tissues.

(4) Nervous tissues.

(5) Reproductive tissues.

EPITHELIAL TISSUE

It is found throughout the body. Epithelial tissue acts as an external layer on the body and around the organs and also forms the internal lining of the organs called the 'mucous membranes.' They serve important functions like protection e.g. skin, secretion e.g. various glands like pancreas, salivary glands or the intestinal glands, absorption e.g. digestive tract or the renal tubules or the inner lining of the heart and blood vessels.

CONNECTIVE TISSUE

Connective tissues are the most widespread tissues in the body. They serve to connect and support organs as well as form the packing substance in between the other tissues and organs. They connect other tissues to each other, connect muscles to muscles, muscles to bone or bone to bone. They consist of widely spread cells which are scattered in a non-living matrix. There are different types of proteins found in the connective tissues:

- ✧ Elastin protein confers elasticity to these tissues.
- ✧ Collagen protein gives strength.
- ✧ Reticular fibre proteins give support.
- ✧ White blood cells, lymphocytes and macrophages which are cells giving immunity against infections.

Some of these connective tissues get ossified by deposition of Calcium Phosphate in the non-living matrix. This leads to bone formation. In certain places, the connective tissue at the ends of these bones contain a gelatine like substance called Chondrin which imparts compressibility. This leads to cartilage formation. Cartilage in ears and nose contain more of elastin protein fibres, hence they are elastic. Certain cartilages have more collagen fibres in them and hence, they are more tough and fibrous. These occur in the form of spinal disks in between vertebrae. The ends of the bones contain cartilages having dense collagen fibres and these form the structure of weight-bearing surfaces of the bones e.g. knee joint. Tendons connect muscles to bones. The connective tissue of the muscle sheath continues up to the connective tissue sheath of the bone (periosteum) in the form of a tendon. Ligaments are other kinds of connective tissue which connect bone to bone and also, form part of the joint capsule.

As these connective tissues have a non-living background matrix and have a poor blood supply, very little healing takes place if they are damaged. Hence, surgery is usually needed for ligament and tendon tears.

BLOOD

Blood is also a form of connective tissue as it connects all the organs of the body and has blood cells suspended in a liquid known as plasma.

MUSCLE TISSUE

Muscle tissue comprises almost 43% of the body tissues in a healthy and lean male and 37% in female. Muscle tissue has certain unique qualities: they can get excited and electrically charged in response to nervous stimuli and they can contract i.e. shorten. There are about 620 muscles in the human body. Their main function is contraction and along with bones, produce motion. They are of two types, voluntary muscles and involuntary muscles. Voluntary muscles are skeletal muscles which can contract according to the individual's wishes. They are directly under the control of the brain and the spinal cord. Involuntary muscles are under the control of the autonomic nervous system and work accordingly e.g. muscles of the digestive tract and the ureter which brings urine from the kidneys to the urinary bladder. Gall bladder contraction is also an example of involuntary muscle contraction. Cardiac muscle exhibits involuntary contraction but, its rate and strength of contraction can be influenced by physical exercise and emotions.

Exercise physiology is mainly by the application of contraction of the voluntary muscles and manipulation of hormonal responses.

NERVOUS TISSUE

Nervous tissue is found in the brain, spinal cord and the various nerves found throughout the body. It is concerned with control of all the bodily functions. It comprises of three types of cells:

- ✧ Axons which are the nerve cells responsible for transmission of nerve impulses, both sensory and motor (those concerned with movement). They are also associated with memory.

- ✧ Neuroglia are the cells which form the supporting framework of the nervous system and are concerned with providing nutrition to the axons and also, their arrangement.

- ✧ Neurosecretory cells are hormone producing cells found in two areas of the brain, the hypothalamus and the back portion of the pituitary gland.

REPRODUCTIVE TISSUE

This is one of the most important tissues of the human body which is responsible for propagation of the species by reproducing offspring. This tissue is found chiefly in the ovaries in females where it produces the egg also known as the ovum and in the male testis where it produces sperms.

Body systems

Body has many systems which work together in perfect harmony to sustain life. Though each system has its separate functions, they need the co-operation of each other to maintain a healthy body. Nevertheless, for academic purposes, I have classified the various systems as follows:

SKELETAL SYSTEM

This system mainly comprises of the bones and cartilages of the body and is concerned with these important functions:

- ✧ Bones provide support to the body.

- ✧ Bones along with muscle contractions create motion.

- ✧ Bones provide protection to vital organs like the brain, heart and lungs.

- ✧ Bone marrow found in the bones is responsible for blood formation (hemopoesis).

MUSCULAR SYSTEM

Muscular system mainly helps in movements. Moreover, muscles act as a storehouse of proteins and amino acids. They also help in propagation of food in the gut for digestion and absorption and also propagation of urine in the urinary tract for its expulsion from the body. Muscles are classified into voluntary and involuntary muscles. Heart is also a muscle which beats without any external stimulus though rate and force of its contraction is modified by human emotions and physical exercise.

NERVOUS SYSTEM

The brain, spinal cord and the rich plexus of nerves found throughout the body are concerned with the functions of memory, movements and assessment and appropriate action on the sensory inputs from the environment.

RESPIRATORY SYSTEM

The respiratory system consists of the nose, larynx (voice box), trachea (wind pipe), its two divisions known as the bronchi and the lungs. Oxygen is removed from air in the lungs and transported via blood to the body's tissues where the fuels are oxidised and then, the waste product of combustion of carbohydrates and fats namely carbon dioxide is transported back to the lungs via blood and it is exhaled. It is also concerned with voice production (phonation).

CARDIO-VASCULAR SYSTEM

The cardio-vascular system consists of the heart, blood vessels (arteries, veins and capillaries) and the blood. This system is mainly concerned with transportation of nutrients to the tissues and removal of waste products. It is also concerned with regulation of blood pressure, temperature of the body and in providing immunity against invading bacteria and viruses. Hormones are transported via blood to their target organs.

URINARY SYSTEM

The urinary system consists of the following organs: two kidneys, ureters (pipes which transport urine to the urinary bladder), urinary bladder and urethra (the channel by which urine is expelled out of the body). Urine is a medium by which waste products of protein metabolism such as urea, creatinine, ammonia and uric acid get excreted out of the body. Kidneys are also concerned with maintaining water and electrolyte balance of the body and in regulating blood pressure. Many drugs and their metabolic end products are excreted in urine.

REPRODUCTIVE SYSTEM

Reproductive system is concerned mainly with producing offsprings and propagation of species. In the male, the reproductive organs are the testes, the vas deferens (the tube which transports sperms to the seminal vesicles), seminal vesicles (the sacs behind the urinary bladder which store sperms), the prostate gland which is situated just below the bladder and is responsible for secreting fluid which forms the semen), the bulbo-urethral glands which adds alkalinity to the semen so that the sperms survive in the acidic environment of the vagina and the penis which deposits sperms in the vagina.

In the female, reproductive system comprises of two ovaries situated in the lower abdomen which form eggs, the two fallopian tubes which transport the egg to the uterus (fertilisation of egg by the sperm happens in the fallopian tube), the uterus which acts as the place where the fertilised egg is implanted and develops into a baby, the cervix which is the muscular junction between the uterus and the vagina which keeps the baby in the uterus till maturity and the vagina which acts as a receptacle for the erect penis and into which sperms are deposited after ejaculation. The ovaries are also concerned with synthesis of female hormones such as Oestrogen and Progesterone.

ENDOCRINE SYSTEM

Various glands are found in the body. They secrete chemicals known as hormones which are transported via the blood stream to the various organs. These hormones influence the metabolism of the body in various ways as will be seen below.

Pituitary gland: It is located at the base of the brain. It is the master gland of the body as the secretion of hormones by most other glands and organs is influenced by the pituitary. The various hormones secreted by the pituitary are

- ✧ **FSH (Follicle Stimulating Hormone)** stimulates production of sperms and testosterone in males and egg formation and oestrogen secretion in the female.

- ✧ **LH (Luteinizing hormone)** stimulates ovaries to secrete progesterone hormone in females, prepares the uterus for implantation of egg and promotes breast development.

- ✧ **GH (Growth Hormone)** regulates metabolism and stimulates tissue growth.

- ✧ **TSH (Thyroid Stimulating Hormone)** promotes secretion of the thyroid hormone thyroxin and also growth of the thyroid gland.

- ✧ **ACTH (Adreno-Cortico-Tropic Hormone)** stimulates the adrenal glands to secrete stress hormone cortisol and also, stimulates the secretion of aldosterone hormone which regulates water and electrolyte balance in the body.

- ✧ **Prolactin** stimulates milk production in the female breast.

- ✧ **ADH (Anti-diuretic hormone)** regulates water absorption by kidneys and causes the small arteries to contract.

- ✧ **Oxytocin** causes uterine contractions and milk ejection from the lactating breast.

Parathyroid glands are four in number and situated on each of the poles of the thyroid gland. They secrete Parathormone which increases blood calcium levels and decreases blood phosphate levels.

Thyroid gland secretes Thyroxin which increases metabolism.

Adrenal Cortex is the outer layer of the adrenal glands which are located on the superior poles of both kidneys. Adrenal cortex secretes two hormones:

✧ **Aldosterone** which regulates water and electrolyte balance in the body.

✧ **Cortisol** works as a stress hormone and regulates carbohydrate, protein and fat metabolism.

✧ **Adrenal Medulla** secretes Adrenaline, Nor-adrenaline and Dopamine which are stress hormones mainly influencing blood pressure. They also play a role in carbohydrate, protein and fat metabolism in response to stress.

Pancreas is located in the abdomen behind the stomach. It secretes two hormones mainly in response to blood glucose levels:

✧ **Insulin** is a hormone secreted in response to high blood sugar levels. It promotes glucose uptake by the body cells and also decreases potassium and phosphate levels in blood.

✧ **Glucagon** is anti-insulin in its action. It increases blood sugar levels by promoting fats and proteins to be converted to carbohydrates. It also increases potassium and phosphate levels in the blood.

Thymus gland is situated in the chest cavity in front of the heart. It secretes a hormone which regulates immunity.

Ovaries are two in number and situated in the lower abdomen on either side of the uterus. The important hormones are oestrogen and progesterone which develop internal and external feminine features.

Testes are two in number and situated in the scrotum. They secrete a hormone known as testosterone which imparts masculine characteristics to an individual. Testosterone is the main hormone in muscle development. All the anabolic and androgenic steroids are testosterone derivatives one way or the other.

These are the different systems of the body which work in an inter-dependent manner to sustain life.

CHAPTER 22

THE MUSCLE

The muscle tissue is the main component on which the entire science of exercises and fitness is based. Muscles comprise almost 43–45% body weight in a lean male and about 32–35% body weight in lean females. Females will tend to have a slightly higher body fat percentage than males and that is natural. There are mainly 620 muscles in the human body. About 20 of them are situated in the eyeball, which help in its movements.

Functions of muscles

(1) **Movement:** Muscles have a property of contraction that is they shorten in length. By this property, they help in movement of the various body parts and also, locomotion.

(2) **Posture control:** By the synchronous contractions of various and at times, opposite muscle groups, muscles help to improve balance and posture.

(3) **Generate heat:** During times of exposure to cold, muscles contract finely with high speeds to produce what is called 'shivering.' This is a mechanism by which heat is generated and prevents the interior of the body to cool down.

(4) **Protection:** A muscular body has less chance of damage during an accident as the big muscles act as cushions and prevent grievous injury.

(5) **Amino acid store:** 80% of the muscle tissue is made up of proteins. This large reservoir of protein can provide a lot of amino acids to synthesize other important proteins in the human body.

Types of muscles

Muscles can be classified into three types mainly based on whether there is voluntary control over the muscle movements.

(1) **Voluntary muscles:** They are mainly found attached to the bones, the eyeball and upper 1/3rd of the foodpipe. They are under the control of the person's mind and work according to the thoughts and desires of the individual. They are also called striated muscles or multinucleate muscles based on their appearance under the microscope but, this is of little relevance here.

(2) **Involuntary muscles:** They are mainly found in the walls of organs, blood vessels and also, under the hair of the skin. They help in forward movement of the contents of the organs e.g. food in the digestive tract or urine in the ureters (the pipes which bring urine from the kidneys to the bladder). In the blood vessels, especially the arteries, they contract to narrow their diameter and relax to enlarge the diameter. This regulates blood pressure. The contraction of muscles under the hair on the skin leads to what is known as 'goose flesh.' The exact importance of goose flesh is unknown in humans. They are also called 'smooth muscles' because of their appearance under the microscopic magnification, but again it is of little relevance here.

(3) **Cardiac muscle:** Cardiac muscle is an involuntary muscle which beats at the rate of 60 – 120 times per minute on its own without the control of the person's mind. Though heart rate is also dependent on the person's emotions and physical exercise, it is purely the hormones of stress namely adrenaline that lead to an increase in the heart rate.

Mechanics of muscle contraction

This section mainly deals with the skeletal muscles which are voluntary. The nerve fibres from the brain activate the neurons (nerve cells) in the spinal cord. The spinal neurons generate an electrical pulse which travels down the nerves to the muscles. Each nerve fibre branches off and supplies many muscle cells (let's call them fibres for the sake of simplicity). The tiny electrical pulse is amplified at its junction with the muscle fibre and it electrifies the surface of the entire muscle fibre. Each muscle fibre is filled with small protein fibrils (tiny fibres) of two different kinds – Actin and Myosin. Upon receiving the electric charge from the nerve, there is a large release of calcium within the muscle cell. This generates another chemical signal and the actin and myosin fibres slide in between themselves, thus shortening the muscle fibre. These muscles are attached by means of connective tissue ropes called tendons to the bones. There are specialised cells present at the junction between the muscle and the tendon which regulate the tension generated by the muscle. It is the combination of muscle contraction and the tension developed which causes movement of the bones and as a result, the body.

Types of muscle contractions

Muscle contraction does not always mean that the muscle will shorten in length. As discussed previously, there are two components of muscle contraction namely developing tension and shortening of the muscle. Now, imagine that you are lifting a heavy weight. At first, you might strain, your muscles will contract but, the weight will not lift. This contraction when the tension increases within the muscle but, the muscle does not shorten is known as '**Isometric contraction.**' Now, if you decrease the weight and try to lift it, it starts budging and you lift it. The tension is of course increased in the muscle but, it remains constant throughout the muscle contraction that is shortening of the muscle. This contraction of the muscle in which the tension in the muscle remains same throughout the movement but, it changes its length is known as '**Isotonic contraction.**' Isotonic contractions can be of two types. Imagine the muscle shortening when you lift the weight. This is known as '**Positive contraction**' and the phase is known as the '**Concentric phase of contraction.**' Now, you start lowering the weight slowly under control. You are in full control over the weight that is being lowered. Your muscle will be under tension and remain partially contracted throughout the lowering phase, but the muscle will gradually lengthen. This is known as '**Negative contraction**' and the phase is referred to as '**Eccentric phase of contraction.**'

Functional classification of muscle fibres

Classification based on the contractile characteristics of the muscle is very important in planning workouts and nutrition of an individual.

TYPE I SLOW-TWITCH; OXIDATIVE; RED MUSCLE FIBRES

This group of muscle fibres are suited for endurance kind of activities like marathons. These muscle fibres are slow-twitch muscle fibres meaning they do not contract explosively. They are usually smaller in diameter, highly resistant to fatigue and have very little capacity for hypertrophy i.e. increase in size. They respond to higher repetitions with lesser weights. Witness the muscles of marathon runners.

TYPE II FAST-TWITCH; OXIDATIVE-GLYCOLYTIC; WHITE MUSCLE FIBRES

This group of muscle fibres are suited for heavy, explosive kind of activities like sprinting, weight lifting, shotput, discus throw etc. They are usually bigger in diameter than the red muscle fibres and have the capacity for further hypertrophy. They respond to higher weights and lesser repetitions. They have the tendency to fatigue easily because of the nature of their metabolism, as lactic acid builds up in them during repetitive contractions and causes fatigue. We will discuss about the energy systems of the muscles in a later chapter. Witness the muscles of sprinters and compare them to the muscles of marathoners.

Based on the above classification of muscles, we will deal with how best they can be developed scientifically with logically engineered workouts and diet plans. After all, it is better to work hard and smart rather than just slogging hard, isn't it?

THINK SCIENTIFIC! BE SCIENTIFIT!

CHAPTER 23

ENERGY SYSTEMS WITHIN THE MUSCLE

Food whether in the form of carbohydrate, protein or fat is primarily composed of carbon, hydrogen, oxygen and nitrogen. Molecular bonds in the macronutrients are relatively weak and energy is released when they are broken down. This energy is not directly used for body functions. Rather there is a very efficient system in the body which traps this released chemical energy in the form of ATP (Adenosine Triphosphate). We had seen earlier that ATP is the energy currency of the body. Whenever energy is needed, this ATP gets broken down to ADP (Adenosine Diphosphate) and a phosphate.

At rest, the body derives energy from the breakdown of carbohydrate and fat. Proteins are the building blocks of the body and they are usually not used for energy production. During moderate to severe muscular effort, more and more carbohydrate is used for energy production and less reliance is put on fat metabolism. In an all-out maximal or sub-maximal effort, energy is derived almost exclusively from carbohydrates.

Carbohydrates

Carbohydrate is stored in the body exclusively in the form of glycogen which is a long chain of chemically bonded glucose molecules. Glycogen is stored in the liver and the skeletal muscles. Glycogen stored in the muscles is not used for energy production elsewhere but, is localised only to that muscle where it is stored. It is the liver that provides blood glucose which is used by various organs for their functions.

The glycogen stores in the body are limited (about 400–500 grams only). This can provide up to 2000 kcal. of energy. Now, the glycogen stored in a particular muscle will be utilised exclusively by that muscle only. Hence, it can be said that the carbohydrate stores in the body need to be replenished from time to time.

The glycogen is stored in the cytoplasm of the liver and muscle cells. They are first broken down to glucose molecules which are further split into pyruvate molecules. Now, the fate of the pyruvate molecules depend on whether adequate oxygen is available during the energy need. When the exercise is done in the presence of a continuous supply of oxygen as in any endurance sport such as jogging, cycling etc. this pyruvate enters the chemical reaction known as 'Krebs Cycle' and forms more molecules of ATP. Compare this to a high intensity sport such as a 100 meters dash. The effort is near-maximal and the availability of oxygen to the tissues is relatively less. In this case, pyruvate is converted to lactic acid in the muscle. This leads to a decreased conversion of glycogen to glucose and further production of ATP. This is the very reason why fatigue sets in very rapidly after a maximal or near-maximal physical effort.

Fats

Fat is said to provide energy about 9 kcal per gram. It is the major fuel used in prolonged low-intensity exercise such as endurance sports. The triglycerides are the fats which provide energy. The process is slightly complex. A triglyceride molecule is first broken down to glycerol and three fatty acids. These fatty acids are further cleaved into a smaller chemical known as acetyl CoA which enters the Krebs cycle and undergoes all the chemical reactions needed to form ATP, carbon dioxide and water. This is a slower process than carbohydrate metabolism and requires oxygen. The chemical combustion of fat is also known as B-oxidation. This combustion of fats yields much higher calories than carbohydrates, but it is a slower process and not so efficient in providing instant energy bursts.

Proteins

Proteins as fuel provide less than 5% of the total calories. Before being burnt off as fuel, proteins should first be converted to glucose by a chemical process called 'Gluconeogenesis.' Proteins can also be used to generate free fatty acids which can either be used as energy sources or are stored as fat. During periods of intense starvation, conversion of proteins into a fuel source takes place. Only the amino acids can be used in this way and yield 4 kcal per gram of protein.

Bioenergetics and dynamics of energy production during muscle contractions

An ATP molecule is composed of one molecule of adenosine, one sugar ribose and three inorganic phosphate groups. When acted upon by the enzyme ATPase, this molecule is cleaved into one molecule of ADP and one phosphate group and a large amount of energy is released as a result of the breakdown of this chemical bond. During intense muscle contractions, almost all the ATP stores in the muscle fibre get depleted within the first 2–3 seconds. For further intense contractions to occur, these ATP stores need to be regenerated. This occurs by three methods in the muscle cell:

(1) **Creatine Phosphate:** All of the gym goers must have come across the supplement Creatine. It is this same creatine that we are talking about. There is a store of creatine phosphate present within the muscle. This is chemically broken down to creatine and phosphate and this phosphate then combines with ADP to reform ATP. There is enough store in the muscle to replenish ATP and continue the high intensity activity for another 8–10 seconds.

(2) **The Glycolytic system:** This is another method which involves the production of ATP from breakdown of Glucose within the cells (Glycolysis). Glucose is stored in the muscle in the form of glycogen. For further ATP molecules, this glycogen is rapidly broken down to glucose molecules by a chemical process called 'Glycogenolysis.' This glucose is further broken down to pyruvic acid. This breakdown does not require oxygen. But, in the absence of oxygen (anaerobic metabolism), this pyruvic acid is converted to lactic acid which accumulates in the muscle and prevents further

breakdown of glycogen to glucose. This energy system yields very less ATP molecules, but, it continues to fuel the intense muscular contractions till the lactic acid stops the process.

(3) **The Oxidative system:** This is the most complex of the three energy systems. The process by which fuel combustion happens in the presence of oxygen is known as 'cellular respiration.' It generates a lot of molecules of ATP and occurs within the mitochondria which is an organelle found in the cells. Unlike anaerobic energy production, the aerobic (in presence of oxygen) system has a tremendous energy producing capacity, so aerobic metabolism is the primary source of energy production during the endurance events.

Based on these backgrounds, it will be easy to understand how exercise and nutritional principles go hand in hand in development of a sound physique and optimum physical performance.

CHAPTER 24

HOMEOSTASIS AND METABOLISM

The body procures nutrients for growth, maintenance, energy, repair and for sustaining life. To accomplish these functions, there are innumerable chemical reactions taking place in the body that occur synchronous to each other so that the end result falls within a desired range. The human body comprises of trillions of cells which together form various tissues, organs and organ systems. These systems are tightly interwoven so that a balance is maintained in the body. There are various physiological mechanisms in the body that are self-regulating in maintaining their rate of chemical reactions to keep the body in a state of perfect equilibrium. Hormone production, maintenance of heart rate and blood pressure within the desired range, regulation of body temperature and regulation of body's fluid and electrolyte balance are some of the examples how our body maintains this equilibrium.

Homeostasis

Homeostasis refers to the chemical processes that maintain the body in a state of constant physiological equilibrium. A superb example of homeostasis mechanism is regulation of body temperature. If the body is exposed to a hot environment, then sweating occurs to cool the body's surface temperature. The blood vessels under the skin open up to dissipate the body heat, hence the flush is felt when exposed to sun. Whenever the body is exposed to cold temperatures, shivering happens to produce that extra heat to raise the body's temperature. Remarkable, isn't it!

Some different homeostatic mechanisms found in the body are as below:

(1) Control of body temperature by shivering and sweating.

(2) Control of the different hormones and their levels in the body.

(3) Maintenance of water and electrolyte balance.

(4) Maintenance of blood glucose levels.

(5) Maintenance of blood gases namely oxygen and carbon dioxide.

(6) Maintenance of acid-base balance in the body.

(7) Maintenance of blood pressure.

(8) Maintenance of fluidity of blood by regulating clotting.

The examples are endless in the human body.

One major example is of interest to us. If you have spent many years in the gym lifting weights, then, your muscles tend to become bigger. They have more contractile myofibrils in them and their ATP and Creatine Phosphate content increases. Their glucose level also increases. This is to counteract the high intensity workouts that the muscles have to endure. Compare this to the individual who takes jogging as a form of exercise. His/her muscles will be small and there will be more of red muscle fibre development. As the muscles of this individual are more tuned to aerobic kind of metabolism, the muscles needn't store a lot of glycogen in them. The fat percentage of these individuals will be higher than that of a sprinter. These muscles will have a higher tendency for aerobic metabolism.

Even nutrition can shift the homeostasis. If you eat more of junk food and fat-rich foods, the homeostasis will shift in such a way that you will gain a lot of body fat. Whereas eating the right kind of food and taking the right kind of supplementation will ensure that you develop the lean muscular look of an athlete. This emphasises the role of nutrition in an individual's life.

Metabolism

In simple terms, metabolism is a process by which the body converts what you eat into growth and energy production. Many different chemical reactions take place to achieve the above goals. Although your metabolism influences your body habitus, it is the quantity and quality of food and also the level of physical activity which determine whether your body will accumulate fat or not.

Broadly, metabolism can be classified into two types:

(1) **ANABOLISM:** When the body assimilates the macronutrients into repair and growth of tissues, the process is referred to as 'anabolism.' Your body will be in a state of 'Positive Nitrogen balance' (refer to the chapter on proteins). This happens during puberty, pregnancy, bulking phase in bodybuilding, healing from major injuries etc.

(2) **CATABOLISM:** When the body is in 'Negative Nitrogen balance,' that is it is in a state of breakdown, the metabolic phase is termed as 'Catabolism.' This happens during starvation, major injuries, burns, eating very little protein which leads to muscle breakdown etc.

FACTORS INFLUENCING METABOLISM

(1) Sex: Males tend to have a slightly higher metabolism than females.

(2) Body type (we will refer to this in a later section).

(3) Hormones.

(4) Physical activity.

(5) Nutrition.

(6) Body composition and musculature.

As you can see, other that the first factor, rest of everything is variable and is modifiable.

Basal metabolic rate (BMR)

Body needs to expend some energy in order to keep its vital functions going. Even when you are at rest, your body needs energy for its basic functions like breathing, circulation of blood, temperature regulation, hormonal activity and repair and growth of tissue. This energy expenditure is said to be the 'basal metabolic rate' of that individual. All the above factors that influence metabolism also influence the BMR.

Other than this, your body requires energy for two more purposes:

(1) Thermogenesis: Food ingested is digested, absorbed, transported and assimilated into tissues and that needs calories. The metabolism suddenly rises after a meal and this is known as a'Thermogenic effect of food.' A large protein meal seems to have a higher thermogenic effect.

(2) Physical activity: Any kind of physical activity needs energy other than that used up by the body as its BMR.

How metabolism influences fat gain?

It is very easy to blame your genetics and your metabolism for your fat gain. But, it is not so. Fat gain is the summation of many factors such as your genetic make-up, hormones, sedentary lifestyle, lack of sleep, lack of proper exercise, increased calorie intake along with improper nutrition and stress. It is very rare to see a client whose fat gain is due to slow metabolism due to hormonal diseases like hypothyroidism and Cushing's syndrome. The simple equation is that if you burn fewer calories than your intake, you get fat. If you burn more calories than your intake, ultimately you will lose weight. End of argument!

Physical activity and metabolism

It may not be possible for you to control your metabolism completely, but one look at the different variables that influence your basal metabolic rate shows that it can be regulated to a large extent through physical exercise and proper diet, especially the exercise part. You can increase your metabolism by increasing your muscle mass which will continue to burn calories even at rest. This can be achieved through a judicious combination of weight training and aerobic activities. You can even increase physical activity through minor variations in your lifestyle like taking the stairs instead of the elevators or parking your car at a distance and walking the rest of the way. Even activities such as household work, washing your car and gardening also increase your calories expenditure.

No magic supplement for fat loss

Though different products have been touted in the market as fat loss supplements, remember that it is more hype than fact. Fat burners don't work; they only burn a hole in your pocket but, never in your fat stores unless you follow a well-planned dietary and exercise regimen. And if you eat clean and train hard, why would you need a 'fat burner?'

NO SHORTCUTS IN LIFE AND IN BODYBUILDING!

CHAPTER 25

BODY MASS INDEX (BMI) AND BODY COMPOSITION

Body Mass Index or BMI

BMI or Body Mass Index is a term used by many nutritional companies for marketing their weight loss supplements. Just go to any store which is selling these products and they will first measure your BMI. Now, let us discuss what exactly BMI is and what is its value in fitness.

BMI is a value that is calculated from the body weight and height of an individual. Its formula is as follows:

BMI = weight (in kg)/square of height in meters (metric units).

BMI = 703 X weight (in lbs)/ square of height in inches (US units).

BMI is used to determine whether the person is underweight, normal weight, over-weight, obese or grossly obese. Commonly accepted BMI value ranges are as follows:

Under 18.5 kg/m^2: Underweight.

18.5–25 kg/m^2: Normal weight.

25–30 kg/m^2: Obese.

30 kg/m^2 and above: Grossly obese.

The bottom line is that BMI values are not designed for muscular people. Volume wise, muscle tends to have more weight that fat. Muscle is heavier than fat by 18%. A muscular person has significantly more muscle mass than fat. BMI takes into account the entire weight of the individual and it completely ignores the lean body mass. At the age of 34 years during the peak of his career as an action hero, Arnold

Schwarzenegger had a BMI of close to 31, which is considered to be grossly obese by any standards. But, was he really obese as his BMI stated? No, he was very, very muscular. This proves that BMI is not the gold standard for determining obesity.

A much better assessment of obesity or your leanness is your body fat percentage and your waist measurements. Even the weight of your body is more or less irrelevant. Body fat percentage can be determined by performing investigations for your body composition.

Body composition

In fitness, you must mould and sculpt your body to meet your specific goals. Leanness is best determined by looking in the mirror than your bathroom scale. The height-weight scales and charts are rudimentary guidelines. If you want to know what exactly your body is made up of and how it will respond to diet and training, then you should get your body composition done. And the most important values to see in body composition is body fat percentage and muscle mass.

METHODS TO DETERMINE BODY FAT PERCENTAGE

(1) **SKIN FOLD CALIPERS:** As more than 50% of your body fat is sub-cutaneous that is just under the skin, it follows that thicker the skin fold, more will be the body fat. Readings are taken at multiple areas on the body and body fat percentage is calculated according to these readings. This technique of measuring body fat percentage is portable, inexpensive and can easily be carried out in the field by skilled and experienced personnel.

(2) **UNDERWATER WEIGHING:** This technique is based on the principle that density of fat is lesser than water; hence, a person with more fat will weigh lesser in water (after complete exhalation, of course) than outside of the water. This technique is quite accurate and inexpensive; unfortunately, it is not portable and cannot be carried out in the field.

(3) **BIOELECTRICAL IMPEDANCE:** The principle behind this technique is that water is a good conductor of electricity. Muscle

contains more water than fat. The rate at which your body conducts electricity determines your body fat percentage. This technique is fairly expensive and quite unreliable. Unfortunately, this is the technique which is performed in most of the fat loss centres and the gymnasiums.

(4) **OTHER LABORATORY METHODS:**

✧ DEXA scan is the gold standard in body fat measurements.

✧ Potassium ion measurements.

✧ Ultrasound.

✧ Infra-red light analysis.

✧ Radiographic analysis like CAT scan.

✧ Proton absorptiometry.

✧ Nuclear magnetic resonance.

Somatotypes (Body types)

The way your body looks depends on both the genetics and the environment. There are two words which need explanation here:

(1) Genotype is the set of genes in our DNA which are responsible for a particular trait.

(2) Phenotype is the expression of that trait.

Colour of hair, eyes and height of an individual is not in his/her hands. But, other characteristics like muscularity, athleticism, fitness levels etc. are certainly in the hands of the person. The genetic factor has dominance on your body structure to some extent, but other factors described above depend on your environment (here environment refers to exercise, nutrition and an active lifestyle).

W. H. Sheldon devised a method of classifying a human body into three broad types:

* **Ectomorph:** An individual with a slim and linear body type who is also called a hard-gainer (difficult to put on muscles). These people have a particularly fast metabolism.

* **Mesomorph:** They are the naturally muscular or athletic type.

* **Endomorph:** They are short, pudgy and fat and supposed to have a sluggish metabolism.

Most individuals have a dominant somatotype but, also display the characteristics of the other two. Most elite world class athletes have dominant mesomorphic traits. But, this certainly does not mean that ectomorphs or endomorphs cannot become superior athletes. By a combination of correct prescription of exercises and proper nutritional planning, any somatotype can scale great heights in the field of fitness and sports.

CHAPTER 26

FACTORS INFLUENCING METABOLISM

Metabolism is the set of chemical reactions taking place in the body to sustain life. We have seen that metabolism can be grossly divided into two categories, anabolism and catabolism. Again, to briefly summarize things, anabolism is the set of chemical reactions needed to repair and grow tissues. The raw materials for growth comes from the food that we eat and also, the breakdown products of other chemicals in the body. The net result of anabolism is that new cellular material is made such as enzymes, cell membranes, proteins and even new cells and tissues. The opposite of anabolism is catabolism which causes tissue breakdown. Complex biomolecules are broken down to release energy e.g. carbohydrates and fats. Some of the biomolecules are recycled to form newer molecules and some of the end-products of catabolism are excreted as waste products in urine and faeces. Anti-oxidants, certain phytochemicals and a good diet can offset many effects of catabolism. When catabolic rates are decreased in certain conditions by a proper combination of diet and supplementation, e.g. correct and proper post-workout meal after very strenuous exercise, the net result will be anabolism, which will lead to better muscle growth and performance.

The word metabolism only applies to changes occurring within the cells. A healthy metabolism requires many enzymes, vitamins, minerals and other co-factors to function smoothly. Enzymes are proteins. Take an instance when a certain amino acid which is necessary to form an enzyme is lacking in the diet. That enzyme will not be formed and hence, the biochemical reaction will be blocked. A deficiency of certain vitamin or mineral can block a biochemical reaction and not allow the set of reactions to reach their end point. The body needs thousands of enzymes for metabolism to proceed along a certain line. So, if you are a fitness freak, you better make sure that your diet contains all the necessary nutrients.

Metabolic set point

The human body is run by a set of chemical reactions which are tightly interwoven and run synchronously. Based on your genetics and your environment, the body seeks to maintain a particular rate of metabolism. The average of this rate of metabolism is known as 'metabolic set point.' Metabolic set point depends on many factors including your level of physical exercise and your nutrition. Take a scenario that you are on a low calorie diet. The body's survival software immediately swings into action and decreases its BMR. If you live in a cold climate, the body's metabolism shoots up to maintain your core body temperature. The metabolic set point is set at a higher level. Exercise tends to increase the level of the metabolic set point.

Food and metabolism

Intake of foods which are particularly rich in proteins and carbohydrates increases your metabolism. There is a 'thermogenic effect' of food i.e. the body spends energy in digestion and processing the foods. Food high in protein has a higher thermogenic effect. Certain supplements such as caffeine also increase metabolism and they can be used as thermogenic aids to boost up metabolism. Many people drink strong black coffee or take caffeine in their pre-workout supplements to boost their energy levels and also, stimulate their nervous system.

WHAT IS RESPIRATORY QUOTIENT?

Your body has a variety of fuels to choose from, namely carbohydrates, fats and proteins. At rest, the body burns a mixture of carbohydrates and fats, whereas during intense exercise, body burns predominantly carbohydrates. Aerobic exercise also burns a mixture of carbohydrates and fats. So, how to determine what exactly is your body burning at a given time?

Your body takes in oxygen via the lungs. This oxygen is used up in the combustion chambers of cells called mitochondria. Fuels are burnt in these chambers in presence of oxygen and the energy is trapped in ATP molecules. Carbon dioxide is the waste product which is transported via blood to the lungs where it is given out in the breath. Now, the amount of carbon dioxide formed will be different for carbohydrates, fats and proteins. This is where the concept of Respiratory Quotient comes in the picture and its equation is as follows:

Respiratory Quotient (RQ) = volume of carbon dioxide given out in the breath divided by volume of oxygen inhaled in each breath.

This means that for a given quantity of oxygen, how much quantity of carbon dioxide is produced by the burning of a certain fuel. Carbohydrates have a respiratory quotient of 1.0 and fats have an RQ of 0.7. Proteins have an RQ of 0.8. At rest, body burns a mixture of fats and carbohydrates with very little protein being burnt as fuel (about 10–15% only; they are mainly used as building blocks). The RQ falls somewhere between 0.7–1.0; usually it is 0.8. During very intense physical activity, RQ values shift towards 1.0 as more carbohydrates are burnt off as fuel.

Factors affecting RQ

(1) **Diet:** A diet more in carbohydrates will shift the RQ towards 1.0, whereas a diet high in fats will shift the RQ towards 0.7.

(2) **Physical conditioning:** A well-trained athlete will be using more of fatty acids for energy as compared to an untrained person. So, the RQ will be around 0.7. During exercise, an untrained individual will utilise more of carbohydrates whereas a trained athlete will be using a mixture of fatty acids and carbohydrates. There will be a corresponding shift in RQ.

(3) **Type of exercise:** High intensity exercise utilises more carbohydrates whereas low intensity aerobic exercise utilises more of fatty acids plus carbohydrates coming a close second.

Environment and metabolism

The environment to which your body is exposed also influences your metabolism to a great extent. If you are suddenly exposed to a colder climate, your body starts shivering. Shivering is a series of involuntary muscle contractions which generate heat. Your body's core temperature rises. If you spend time in a colder climate, your metabolism actually rises and your metabolic set point is set at a higher level. Conversely, when you are exposed to a warm climate, your metabolism slows down and metabolic set point shifts to a lower level.

Physical exercise and metabolism

Physical exercise raises your metabolic set point and increases your metabolism even when you are resting. Muscles use up a lot of energy for their maintenance. Even when they are resting, they continue to burn energy. We will see in detail the metabolic changes happening in the muscles as a result of physical training in the next chapter.

CHAPTER 27

EXERCISE PHYSIOLOGY AND METABOLISM

Exercise will set off a lot of metabolic changes in the body which affect its anatomy, physiology and biochemistry. Exercise or any sport event is primarily of two types: explosive and endurance. Examples of explosive exercises are weight training with very heavy weights, shot putting, discus throwing, tennis serve etc. Endurance events mainly comprise long distance running, long distance swimming, cycling etc.

If you remember, during heavy weight lifting or other explosive type of sports, the oxygen supply to the athlete cannot cope up with the increased demand of the exercising muscles. Hence, this type of exercise is also known as anaerobic exercise (insufficient oxygen). In the other type, the intensity of exercise is low to moderate and muscle contractions are even. The explosive phase is rarely used. The oxygen supply to the exercising muscles matches the oxygen demand. The metabolism within the contracting muscle fibres provides a continuous energy source during the event as a result of continuous oxygen supply. This type of physical activity is also known as aerobic activity or aerobic exercise.

Energy metabolism within the exercising muscles

Energy metabolism is a series of chemical reactions taking place in the cell to provide energy to the exercising muscles. It results from the breakdown of foodstuffs like carbohydrates (mainly glucose), fatty acids and sometimes amino acids. About 75–80% of the energy released during this breakdown is in the form of thermal energy and dissipated as heat, hence the increased heat production during exercise. Effectively, only 20–25% of the energy is used for effective muscle contraction. As we have learnt, ATP is the energy currency of the body. It is the breakdown of ATP to ADP and a Phosphate group which yields energy. Whatever foodstuffs are broken down for energy, the target end result is ATP formation. First and foremost, we have to understand that at any given time, a contracting muscle has ATP stores to fuel only the first 2-3 seconds of contractions. For further continuation of contractions, other pathways come into play. For another 10-12 seconds, it is the Creatine Phosphate (CrP) stores which give their phosphate group to ADP and ATP is again regenerated to be used for further activity. When after 12-15 seconds of continued muscle activity when even the CrP stores get depleted, a third chemical reaction kicks in. There are many ADP molecules accumulating in the muscle now. Two molecules of ADP will unite to form one molecule of ATP and one molecule of AMP (adenosine monophosphate). This gives another 2-3 seconds of muscle contractions. If the exercise still continues after that, glycogen present in the cytoplasm of muscle cells breaks down to glucose. One molecule of glucose splits into two molecules of pyruvate and two molecules of ATP are formed in the process. Further metabolism of pyruvate is determined by whether the exercise is anaerobic or aerobic. If it is anaerobic, pyruvate is converted to lactic acid which accumulates in the muscle and inhibits further breakdown of glycogen to glucose, thereby inhibiting any further effective exercise. Lactic acid also causes cramping in the muscles. This lactic acid is then washed away via the blood stream to the liver where it is recycled back to glucose. If the conditions of the exercise is aerobic, pyruvate enters the mitochondria and goes through the Krebs cycle (we read about it earlier) and this forms more ATP molecules than those formed under anaerobic conditions. As a result, intense events are usually terminated early because of cramps and fatigue, whereas aerobic or endurance events last longer, sometimes even up to a few hours.

The type of exercise also affects the anatomy (shape), physiology (workings) and biochemistry (different metabolic pathways) of a muscle. We have already seen that there are two types of muscles, red and white. White muscles are explosive energy generating muscles which contract under anaerobic conditions and are glycolytic. In order to produce more and more powerful contractions, white muscle cells have to pack in more contractile proteins, creatine and glucose. Hence, they grow bigger in size. Aerobic training conditions the red muscle fibres to develop more than white muscle fibres in a particular muscle. They are muscle fibres for endurance which contract with lesser intensity and hence, they do not have to store many contractile proteins in them as well as creatine phosphate and glycogen as they are not conditioned to generate short bursts of explosive energy. Rather, they are conditioned for low intensity sustained type of activity. Hence, they do not grow in size as big as the white muscle fibres. You can easily tell the difference between the muscles of a sprinter and a marathoner.

Energy systems within the muscles

(1) Energy from stored ATP: This energy can be used for immediate all-out effort lasting 1–3 seconds. It generates strength and power. Power-lifting, shot-putting, discus throwing, tennis serve etc. are examples.

(2) Energy from ATP and CrP stores: This energy system fuels about 10–12 seconds of all-out effort that is sustained-power. Sprints, football etc. are examples.

(3) ATP, CrP and Lactic acid pathway: Fuels about 1–2 minutes of anaerobic power-endurance type of activities. 200–400 yards sprint, 100 yards swimming are examples.

(4) Aerobic oxidative energy: This energy system comes into play in aerobic-sustained type of events lasting more than two minutes e.g. long distance running, cycling etc.

Red muscle fibre changes due to aerobic training

(1) Greater development of slow-twitch (red) muscle fibre.

(2) Increased capacity of muscle to metabolise fatty acids as fuel by increasing enzyme production responsible for mobilising fat from fat depots and also, increasing the number of blood vessels to the exercising muscles.

(3) Increased mitochondria in the red muscle fibres for increased aerobic metabolism of fuels.

(4) Increased myoglobin content (The red pigment found in muscles which act as storage and also transporter of oxygen within the muscles.

White muscle fibre changes due to anaerobic training

(1) Increased number of white muscle fibres (fast-twitch).

(2) Increased size of white muscle fibres to accommodate more myofibrils (contractile proteins), ATP, CrP and glycogen within the muscles.

(3) Increased enzymes for glycolysis (splitting of glucose).

(4) Increased tolerance to higher blood levels of lactic acid.

(5) Increased growth hormone and testosterone levels after 45–60 minutes of intense weight training which leads to anabolism (increased muscle growth).

Metabolism of fatigue

The biochemical concepts behind the metabolism of fatigue works in both untrained as well as trained individuals. This emphasises the importance of exercise in our daily routines. You might not be an athlete but, if you exercise then, you can certainly delay the onset of fatigue in your daily life.

Carbohydrates act as fuel for the exercising muscles. Muscles that generate power and strength primarily use glycogen as their main fuel source. Muscles that generate mild-moderate power over a sustained period i.e. endurance activity, utilise mainly fatty acids as fuels, but even in this case, glucose metabolism is a must. In fact, fatty acids cannot be utilised as fuel in absence of glucose. Bearing this in mind, let us see the chemistry of fatigue.

(1) Glycogen depletion in the body and in the exercising muscles.

(2) ATP and CrP depletion.

(3) Lactic acid build up in the muscles and in the blood.

(4) Nerve impulses coming from the brain and spinal cord to the muscles cause lots of calcium ions to be secreted in the muscles. The concentration of calcium increases in the muscle cells after repeated contractions.

(5) Anaerobic metabolism because oxygen is either depleted or because of poor conditioning of the body; less oxygen is being taken in by the lungs and less is being delivered to the tissues.

The entire physiology given in this chapter can be utilised for muscle development and fat loss. Read on.

CHAPTER 28

THE ACTUAL CAUSE OF FAT GAIN!

Obesity epidemic is rampant in the modern society today in spite of numerous fat free food items that abound the shelves of the supermarkets and food stores. Teen obesity is a major problem today. Numerous theories have been propounded for the same. I only say one thing: if these theories are correct, then performing the reverse of what is mentioned in them should lead to significant fat loss. But, it usually does not happen. Many theories say that sedentary lifestyle leads to obesity. But, we have seen very active individuals who are grossly obese. So, is it only the daily activity of a person or eating more calories than the person's maintenance quota that leads to fat gain? Or whether the source of the calories is also important? Let us logically see why fat gain occurs.

Imagine a container holding water. The amount of water held in that container will be limited. Now, pour extra water in that container. What happens? The water spills out.

Keeping the above example in the forefront, and based on the logical understanding what we have acquired in the previous chapters the concept of fat gain will be very clear to you.

Excess carbohydrate as the culprit

Our body has a limited store of carbohydrates which are stored in the muscles and liver. An average person holds about 400-500 grams of glycogen in the body. Now, most of our diets are carbohydrate rich. What happens is that we periodically eat our meals throughout the day whether we are hungry or not. The carbohydrate stores in our body never have the chance to empty. They are always nearly full. Whenever we eat a high carbohydrate meal, insulin is released by the pancreas. There is one main action of insulin and that is decrease in blood sugars. Now, if the carbohydrate stores in the body are full and we have eaten a carbohydrate rich meal which we usually do, what happens? Insulin gets released. This excess carbohydrate has to go and deposit somewhere. Its designated stores are full. Hence, carbohydrates have no other option but, to get converted to fat and stay deposited in the fat stores.

Now, think again. Most of our diets are rich not only in carbohydrates, but also in fats. Where do you think this excess fat is going? In non-exercising individuals, body utilises more carbohydrates than fats. All this excess fat is deposited in fat stores.

What happens in non-exercising individuals? Here, inactive refers to those individuals who have a primary desk job and who do not have to move about much for their normal activities. Their energy requirements are very less and their intake is more. Excess calories get deposited as fats.

Some very active individuals are also obese. More active an individual, more he/she eats throughout the day the wrong kinds of food and more is the tendency for obesity as mentioned above.

Some of the clients what we see in the gym are obese. They might be able to lift weights, but they are obese. Their minds are hammered by the so-called trainers that if they eat more protein, they will become more muscular. It is very common to find such people gobbling proteins at every opportunity and drinking protein shakes throughout the day. Each body needs a particular amount of protein for its daily needs, growth and also, to remain fit. If excess protein is eaten more than what the body needs, it gets translated to obesity.

One very important factor that leads to obesity needs to be mentioned here. If your food is containing more of high glycemic carbohydrates that is fast digesting carbohydrates, the blood sugar levels tend to rise faster and higher because glucose rapidly enters the bloodstream. Hence, the insulin secretion will also be higher. The glucose load will rapidly rise in the body giving the body insufficient time to direct it to the appropriate organs and then, this glucose will be re-directed towards fat formation. Hence, it is advisable to avoid sweets and processed foods with high glycemic carbohydrates whenever you want to lose fat.

Fat cells are round spherical cells found everywhere in the human body. The fat gets deposited in these cells which swell initially and then, divide. Now, if an obese person loses fat, then his fat cells shrink but, do not decrease in number. But, during the process of development of obesity, the fat cells do increase in number. So, there are more number of cells that can store fat in an obese individual who has lost fat. As these depots have only shrunk in size but, are still present in great numbers, an obese person who with great effort is able to lose fat should be very careful in life with his/her dietary habits and physical exercises because he/she has a higher chance of getting fat again.

The chief causes of obesity

(1) The most indisputable fact is that if your calories intake is more than your output, then you will gain fat. The excess calories may be in the form of carbohydrates, fats, proteins or alcohol.

(2) Eating food rich in carbohydrates and fats, more than what your body needs.

(3) A sedentary lifestyle.

(4) Eating high glycemic index foods.

(5) Certain medical conditions which, if untreated, may lead to obesity.

Role of genetics in obesity

It is generally said and accepted that obesity is genetic. If your parents are fat, then you have a natural tendency to be fat. This argument does not hold true always. Even if you have the genes, how they are expressed is in your hands. Remember the topic on genotype and phenotype. It is very easy to blame the genes even if the fault lies within you. You tend to acquire eating habits from your parents; you inherit their sedentary lifestyle and then, you blame the genes. The truth is that when you modify your lifestyle, then obesity can be prevented. It is like this; you cannot change the colour or texture of your hair but, giving it a certain style is well within your reach.

REMEMBER, OBESITY DOES NOT RUN IN THE FAMILY. IT IS BECAUSE NO ONE RUNS IN THE FAMILY.

CHAPTER 29

THE FALLACY OF STARVATION DIETS

The most common scenario

An obese person goes to a weight loss clinic. He/she is referred to a dietician. The client is prescribed a diet which is extremely low caloric and usually doesn't have a proper macronutrient ratio. It causes rapid weight loss initially which is glycogen and water loss. The client is very happy for the first two days but, then gradually starts feeling severe weakness and fatigue. The weight loss happens maybe in the first week after which it stagnates. The client goes back to the dietician who further drops the calories in the diet. Again (if the client is lucky), weight loss begins and then, again plateaus off. By this time, the client is ravenous and craves to eat. Weakness abounds. The family of the client persuades him/her to start eating again because weight loss is not the only thing that is important in the client's life, there are other important businesses to attend to such as earning the livelihood. This particular starved client will inevitably overeat and regain all the weight that was lost. In many cases, the weight regained is much more than the weight lost.

Another scenario

The client joins a gym in the hope of getting slim and lose weight. The trainers will invariably put such a client on a treadmill and ask to walk at a steady pace whichever is comfortable to the client. I fail to understand that if you have to walk on a treadmill, then why join a gym? Walk in the open. That might not make you fit but, it will save you a lot of money. Just go to a gym and you will see all the obese people there on the treadmills. Go back to the same gym after a few months and you will notice the very same people on the treadmills but, this time with much more body fat.

Then, where are we going wrong?

The default software of the human body

Let us understand the concept behind the programming of the human body. The human body has a built-in software by default and that software is 'SURVIVAL.' Many people survive after major accidents or illnesses. Our body has a tremendous capacity for healing and survival. Over the centuries, humans have faced famines and starvations very frequently. Hence, the body has acquired this particular software by the evolutionary process. It sees fat depots as assets (a very big store house of energy) which it can use in times of starvation. Hence, the body will try to preserve the fat depots as much as it can at the expense of lean body mass. We saw in the previous chapter that body has to spend energy to grow muscles and to maintain them. So, for the body, muscles are liabilities. So, what will the body do under conditions of starvation as with a dietician's diet? I hope the picture is clear to you.

Metabolism and Basal Metabolic Rate revisited

Our body burns carbohydrates, fats and only under extreme conditions the proteins. It utilises this energy for its various functions and also for growth and maintenance. This is known as metabolism. Now, imagine a body at complete rest, though not sleeping. It will still be breathing and its heart will still be beating. The lungs will be working, also the brain, liver and the kidneys. It has to regulate its blood pressure and temperature. It has to fight the bacteria and viruses entering it. The body burns a certain amount of calories to maintain itself in this basal state. This is known as 'Basal Metabolic Rate.' Other activities of the body like walking, talking, working, exercise etc. will consume additional calories.

Under resting conditions, body burns carbohydrates and fats to maintain its various functions. During intense activities like heavy work and heavy exercise, body burns primarily carbohydrates.

What exactly happens in Starvation?

Our body has a limited store of carbohydrates. An average male will be holding 400-500 grams of glycogen in his skeletal muscles and the liver. Imagine now that this same person is given a diet which is much lower in calories than his BMR. The body will initially burn carbohydrates present in it and also some fat. Body has about 2000 calories worth of carbohydrates in it. Each gram of glycogen will hold on to 4 grams of water. So, as soon as these carbohydrate stores are finished, this water loss also occurs. The body will now gradually shift towards burning fats. But, at the same time, the body's survival mechanism becomes auto-activated. The brain is one organ which utilises primarily glucose for its functions. Blood glucose levels drop. Insulin secretion from Pancreas stops. The anti-insulin hormones become active. They try to elevate the blood sugars for the brain to use. Now, the body views the amino acid stores which are present in the muscles' proteins. Certain amino acids can be converted to glucose by a chemical process called 'Gluconeogenesis.' To acquire those amino acids, proteins in the muscles are broken down. These amino acids are converted to glucose in the liver. At the same time, fats are also broken down to form chemicals called 'ketones' which can be used as fuel. So, at this stage it is mainly the muscle proteins which are broken down with some amounts of fats.

So, what happens with low calorie diets?

Whenever an individual starts consuming a low calorie diet with improper ratio of carbohydrates, proteins and fats, the glycogen stores in the body are rapidly exhausted. Around 2 litres of water is also lost along with this glycogen. Bingo! You have a weight loss of about 2-3 kilograms in the first two days and you are very happy. Now, the body turns towards its amino acid stores in the muscles. The muscles rapidly get wasted with very little fat loss. As the person is consuming very little calories with obviously very little amount of proteins, the weight loss will be rapid initially with lot of muscle proteins getting broken down. Body fat percentage actually increases. One other very important source of this initial fast weight loss is that as food intake is very less, the intestines rapidly evacuate their contents as faeces, but after that very little faeces are formed. With some of the meal replacement liquid diets available in the market nowadays, there is hardly any fibre in the meals which will form new stools. Even this is seen as weight loss.

Why does 'Weight loss' stall?

I mentioned before that in response to decreased intake of calories, the body drops its BMR. The body starts using lesser calories for its maintenance. It decreases and sometimes even shuts down some of its functions. The individual does not have the energy to perform vigorous activities and hence, such activities are avoided. A stage comes when the BMR is so low that it exactly balances the daily calories eaten. Hence, the weight loss nearly stalls.

How is the weight regained once normal diet is resumed?

The BMR of an individual has dropped to a low level. Weight loss stalls. The client gets frustrated by such a low calorie diet in which there is perpetual hunger. He/she resumes eating. The calories in the daily diet increases. BMR is very low at this point. Whatever calories are eaten by the client are far in excess to the requirements as BMR is very low. So, all the excess calories do not have a choice but, to go to the fat depots. So, at the end of a total dieting interval, the client has lost a significant amount of muscle and gained a significant amount of fat.

WHAT KIND OF STUPID DIETING PLANS ARE THESE?

GENERAL MOTORS DIET is a very glamorous but a perfect example of an imperfect diet plan.

There must be a way to lose pure fat and still retain all your lean body mass. Yes, there is!

CHAPTER 30

BALANCED DIET IS A MYTH; QUANTIFIED DIETS ARE THE REALITY

What is a balanced diet?

When people hear the word 'diet' what comes to mind is severe restriction of calories or severe restriction of fat intake. Most of us are overwhelmed with conflicting nutritional and dietary advices perpetuated by these so-called 'dieticians' and 'nutritionists,' but, one thing that I have learnt both theoretically and in hundreds of my clients is that deprivation of food is not the solution. It is essential to get the right type and amount of foods in your body in order to achieve a healthy lifestyle.

I totally disagree with the 'Balanced Diets' prescribed by dieticians. They have laid down certain principles which state that diet should have 60% of calories coming from carbohydrates, 25% from proteins and 15% from fats. Each literature and each dietician have their own skewed up ratio. They have also given the food items that are to be eaten under the heading of different macronutrients such as carbohydrates, proteins and fats. My contention is that when the body type of each one of us is different, the body composition, daily activities and the dietary habits of each one of us is different, how can there be a universal balanced diet for all? I am not thinking in an extraordinary manner. This is simple logic, and that is what is lacking in the minds of the experts today.

What are Quantified Diets?

Healthy lifestyle for some people means losing fat, for some it means building muscle and for some means having an abundance of energy to fulfil their vocational and leisure tasks with ease. Each of these lifestyle goals are unique and so is the individual. We have already explained the different somatotypes or body types of individuals such as ectomorphs, mesomorphs or endomorphs. Each of them have a different pattern of metabolism. Each of us fall somewhere in between these categories. The metabolic needs of each one is different. For example, an ectomorph can burn off the calories even if majority of them come from carbohydrates. If you give the same amount of carbohydrates to an endomorph, the individual will put on a lot of fat in no time. One person has time for workouts in the morning, another has time during the day and someone works out in the evening. How can their dietary needs be the same?

CALCULATIONS OF QUANTIFICATION

When a person comes for a diet plan, the parameters that are to be seen are the age, gender, height, weight and body composition (especially the fat percentage). The next thing you ask for are the activities that are performed by the person during an ordinary day. You ask the person the time of waking up, time of sleep and the time when the subject will exercise (if the person exercises at all). Next, you and your client should sit together and determine his/her goal, whether it involves fat loss, whether it involves muscle gain, whether it involves being fit or whether it is just a maintenance diet. The basal metabolic rate and the daily activity levels are determined and the calculated calories are exactly split into an appropriate ratio of carbohydrates, proteins and fats which will lead the individual towards his/her goal. This balance will be different in different individuals. When the calories counted are so exact in nature and we are aware of the dietary habits of the individual, especially what food items are cooked in their homes, then an exact estimate of the food items can be given to that person in grams or millilitres and not according to the size of bowls and cups.

Quantified diets are exactly that.

There will be opposition to this theory that is it necessary to measure each food item correctly before eating. Does this ritual have to be followed the entire life? My counter argument to this is that I always advocate a change in the lifestyle which goes on the lines of a correct exercise plan and dietary plan. Why not? You hire an interior designer for your house and the expert gives you guidelines on what to do. Why not have a blueprint for a more important structure that is your own body? If you are indulging in weight training plus cardio till a ripe old age, and you deviate from the diet a few times, that is perfectly okay within reasonable limits. But, it should not be made a habit.

The advantage of quantified diets is that as you have an exact eating plan, there are few margins for error. Try not to cheat on the diet. You can spend a little lesser time on the social media and more time on the internet searching for the nutritional value of certain foods that you commonly eat. Invest a little time on yourself. It will pay you and your dear ones in the long run. After all, your children will take to your eating habits.

And when you are on a very strict diet plan, never cheat. WILFUL CHEATING WHEN ON A DIET IS NOT PERMISSIBLE; IT DOESN'T WORK.

CHAPTER 31

GENERAL MOTORS DIET: A PERFECT EXAMPLE OF AN IMPERFECT DIET PLAN

General Motors diet was developed for the employees of General Motors. This program was developed in conjunction with a grant from U.S. Department of Agriculture and the Food and Drug Administration. This program is available at all General Motors Food Service Facilities. This program is designed for a weight loss of 10–17 lb per week (mind you, it is weight loss, not fat loss). The promotors of this diet felt that it improves the attitude and well-being of the employees and also has a 'systemic cleansing effect.' Then, my question is if the system is clogged with toxins, it means the liver and kidneys are not functioning; what has diet got to do with this? Go and see a Gastroenterologist or a Nephrologist.

So, what is a General Motors Diet?

During the first seven days of the diet, you must not consume alcohol. You must drink at least 10 glasses of water per day.

Day 1: You can eat any fruits except bananas.

Day 2: You should start this day with a large baked potato. Throughout the day, you can eat any steamed vegetables of your choice.

Day 3: You can eat any fruits and steamed vegetables on day three. But, you cannot eat bananas and potatoes.

Day 4: You will eat eight bananas and three glasses of milk. This should be combined with a special General Motors Soup.

Day 5: This is the day when you can eat a lot of meat and tomatoes. You should increase your water intake today.

Day 6: You can eat meat and vegetables up to any quantities.

Day 7: Brown rice, fruits and as many vegetables that you can consume.

GM WONDER SOUP

This soup is intended to be a supplement to the diet and can be consumed in large quantities. Its ingredients are:

- 28 oz. water.
- 6 large onions.
- 2 green peppers.
- Whole tomatoes.
- 1 cabbage.
- 1 bunch celery.
- 4 sachets of Lipton onion mix.
- Herbs and flavouring as desired.

BEVERAGES THAT CAN BE CONSUMED

- Water.
- Soda.
- Black coffee.
- Black tea.
- Fruit juices on day 7.

Dissection of General Motors Diet

Day 1: You are taking only fruits on day 1. Fruits contain fructose which is a slow digesting sugar. Fruits contain a lot of fibre. So essentially, you are taking lesser calories than your requirements and there is no proteins or the essential fats in your diet which the body needs for its daily function, maintenance, repair and growth. Your carbohydrate stores start to dwindle, but they are never empty because you are taking carbs in the form of fruits. Moreover, you are not taking any sodium in the diet.

Day 2: You take a baked potato (complex carbohydrates) in the morning. Early morning is not the time to take complex carbohydrates. Your brain utilises glucose throughout the night and it derives this glucose from the blood. Liver glycogen supplies blood glucose. Fructose if taken in the morning will be processed by the liver to glucose and stored. So, it is always advisable to eat fruits in the morning and not complex carbohydrates as these will replenish muscle glycogen and not liver glycogen. Again, there is no protein or essential fats on day 2. Body starts to burn its muscle protein to meet its protein requirements. Again, no electrolytes in the diet.

Day 3: You again take fruits and vegetables in your diet. No proteins are taken. Body continues burning muscle proteins in response to a hypo-caloric diet. This is your third day without sodium. Your electrolyte balance starts wobbling.

Day 4: You take bananas, milk and soup. Milk contains negligible amounts of proteins. Bananas contain carbohydrates in the form of glucose and fructose. Very negligible proteins and sodium is being taken. Body continues to burn its muscle proteins and some amount of fat, and carbohydrates. Electrolytes become severely depleted.

Day 5: You are allowed meat and tomatoes. I fail to understand why only tomatoes are allowed. Why hold back on the other vegetables? If you need fibre in the diet, then other vegetables will supply them in abundance. Again, it's an example of a low calorie diet with only protein and fibre. Some fat is present in meat and also used during cooking of the meat, but this is not enough. Body will once again try to deplete its carbohydrate stores on day five.

Day 6: You are allowed only meat and vegetables. Again, you are only taking proteins and fibres and not taking any carbohydrates. This is the day when you burn significant fat.

Day 7: You are only eating rice, vegetables and fruit juices. You are replenishing your carbohydrate stores and essentially stopping the burning of your fat stores.

Pitfalls of GM diet

- ✧ No effort is made to eat the essential fats at least for the first four days. Essential fats are a very important macronutrient and need to be taken daily in the right quantities.

- ✧ Protein is only given on day five and six. During rest of the days, there is no protein in the diet. The body dips into its protein stores and muscle protein undergoes catabolism to fulfil the body's daily protein requirements. Suddenly, on day five and six, you take a high amount of protein, thinking that this will replenish the protein stores, but there is no such thing as an instant protein store. You need to take a particular amount of protein daily in order to preserve your muscles and to keep some of your vital functions humming. Eating excess proteins for two days in a week and staying protein-starved for the rest of the week is not the correct approach.

- ✧ Carbohydrates are replenished in some way or the other daily except on days five and six during which they are mainly in the form of fibres. The body's stores of carbohydrates are remaining nearly full so there is no stimulus for the body to burn fat in excess. A little quantity of fat is used as fuel but, not to the extent desired.

Summary

General Motors Diet is a very imperfect diet. The subjects might experience weight loss, but that loss is mainly water loss because sodium intake is very less. Lot of muscle proteins are being burnt five days in a week because of almost nil protein intake. Little amount of fat is also burnt in the process because the diet is a low calorie diet. Instead of the body weight, we should be checking the body fat percentage of the person who is on a GM diet and I am sure it will be seen that it is higher than day one when he/she started the diet.

THINK SCIENTIFIC! BE SCIENTIFIT!

CHAPTER 32

DISSECTION OF ROUTINE INDIAN FOODS

I was thinking a thousand times before writing this article because it involves a very sensitive topic. We are all used to eating 'Ghar Ka Khana' made by our grandmothers, mothers and wives which includes chapattis, vegetables (either in the form of dry preparations or in form of curry), dal and rice. Our special and exotic foods include paneer (a special kind of cheese), rajma (kidney beans), Chana (chickpeas) etc. And many of us are used to having sweets as desserts at the end of the meal.

Have you ever thought why we Indians are so backward when it comes to sports as compared to athletes of other countries? True, we have our share of 'Pehelwans' or wrestlers but, look at their physique. They have more fat on their body as compared to muscle. Ever thought why?

Nutritional value of 'Ghar ka Khana'

Let us now understand the nutritional value behind the standard 'Ghar ka khana.' Chapattis are made from wheat. And wheat contains fast-digesting carbohydrates. Wheat does contain a protein known as 'Gluten,' but it is found in very less quantities. And a very few of us are 'gluten sensitive.' Will eating chapattis 3-4 times in a day really fulfil your protein requirements?

Our vegetable preparations which are fried in ghee or oil (most of us use oil) are a mixture of negligible amounts of carbohydrates, fibres and fat. Again, extremely low amounts of protein!

Rice is again a rich source of carbohydrates, though it contains protein in small amounts. And Dal, even if it contains proteins, is primarily composed of carbohydrates. The proteins in the Dal have very low biological value.

The more exotic Indian dishes

Let us focus on the more exotic Indian dishes that all of us relish. 'Pavbhaji,' for instance is a good example of carbohydrates, fats and fibre. And what about 'Makki ki roti and Sarson ka saag?' Huge amount of carbohydrates and fibre with added dollops of butter containing a lot of fat. Also, take the Paneer varieties for instance. Paneer contains lot of fat and good amount of protein, but the fat content is much more. And Paneer is usually cooked in a gravy containing dry fruits or 'Khoya' which contains a rich amount of fat.

Indian food has mainly focussed on taste rather than its nutritional value. My one question to all the Indian food lovers is: "Where is the protein?"

An average 65 kg person needs minimum 70 grams of proteins to survive well. And to live a fit lifestyle, the protein intake has to be much more than this. Are we really taking that much protein?

Some people take milk as a source of protein and feel quite contended about it. Just look up the nutritional value of milk on the internet. 100 ml milk contains 3.5 grams of carbohydrates, 3.5 grams of protein and 3.0 grams of fat. How many litres of milk do you think you have to drink daily to fulfil your protein requirements?

All of us love fruits and consider them to be a healthy alternative to meals. It is a fact that fruits contain vitamins but, more amounts of vitamins and minerals can be obtained by eating green leafy vegetables at a much lower cost. Fruits contain fibres but, more fibres are obtained in the vegetables minus the huge amount of carbohydrates in the fruits.

Do you realise now why obesity and diabetes type II along with its accompanying complications like heart attacks and strokes are on an increase in India?

There are some very good food combinations like fish curry and rice eaten in some regions of India. This dish is a perfect example of a good combination of carbohydrates, proteins and healthy fats. Fish curry can also be replaced by chicken curry or mutton curry. But, again try not to make calorie dense gravies like butter chicken or mutton masala. Eating high quantities of fats with high quantities of carbohydrates is like inviting obesity over to dinner.

A good, balanced and healthy source of macronutrients are to be found in dishes such as baked rajma (kidney beans) or Kabuli Chana (chick peas). These items contain balanced amounts of carbohydrates along with high quantity of fibre and good quality proteins. Sprouts are also good examples of good quality proteins admixed with fibre and some carbohydrates. And if you are a non-vegetarian, then eating tandoori or grilled food along with salads is a very good option.

I sincerely hope that I have not offended anyone. But, truth has to be told.

CHAPTER 33

DIABETES MELLITUS TYPE II: WHY INDIA IS RACING AHEAD OF OTHER COUNTRIES?

Diabetes mellitus is a chronic condition that affects your body's ability to utilise carbohydrates as fuel. There are three major types of diabetes: type I, type II which is a lifestyle disorder (according to me) and Gestational Diabetes (occurs in pregnancy and sometimes, stays forever).

Diabetes mellitus type I

This is also called insulin-dependent diabetes or juvenile-onset diabetes as it often occurs in youth. This type of diabetes usually affects young adults. It is an auto-immune condition, meaning that the body's immunity (defence system against bacteria and viruses) starts to attack and destroy its own cells (in this case, the beta cells present in the pancreas). This greatly decreases the pancreas' ability to produce insulin in response to rising blood sugar levels after a meal. This insulin drives the glucose and amino acid molecules in the cells of the body. Absence of insulin often leads to a rapid rise in blood glucose levels, but the body is not able to utilise the glucose for its energy requirements. This is like a thirsty person in the middle of the ocean (poverty in plenty). The blood sugar levels often rise to toxic proportions (hyperglycaemia). More sugar is lost in urine and draws a lot of water along with it, hence urine is passed in excess (polyuria). To compensate for this, the patient's thirst mechanism gets over-activated and leads to increased water consumption (polydipsia). The body cannot utilise carbohydrates as fuel. Hence, the counter-regulatory hormones of the body come into excess play and the body turns to its protein and fat stores for energy.

Excessive catabolism of muscles and fat occurs leading to a rapid decrease in the person's weight. To mobilise the fat stores for energy, the enzyme 'Lipase' becomes over-active in the fat cells and this splits the fat molecules into glycerol and fatty acids. These fatty acids travel to the liver where they are further broken down into 'ketones.' Ketone levels rise in the blood and when combined with hyperglycaemia, leads to a state of 'Ketoacidosis' in which the blood becomes excessively acidic. This can lead to what is called as 'Diabetic Coma,' which can be fatal in the absence of insulin replacement therapy.

Diabetes mellitus type II

Diabetes mellitus type II begins later in life (usually around the age of 40 years) and accounts for almost 95% of the cases. In this type, there is usually an insulin-resistant state, hence blood sugars tend to be elevated. The body initially compensates by secreting more insulin to control the blood sugars, but, the resistance overcomes the insulin concentration in the blood and blood sugars continue to rise. Most people with diabetes type II are obese with a lot of sub-cutaneous and intra-abdominal fat. Onset is usually accompanied by non-specific symptoms such as blurred vision, poor wound healing and vaginal infections.

Diabetes type II presents in four stages:

(1) Stage I: Insulin sensitivity is reduced. Increased insulin levels are present in the blood (hyperinsulinemia) to compensate for the insulin resistance in the body and blood sugars are borderline elevated. There is normal or borderline glucose tolerance test. It is believed that there is a genetically related defect in glycogen synthesis in the skeletal muscles. This disease then gradually progresses to stage two.

(2) Stage II: There is impaired glucose tolerance and relative insulin insufficiency. Random blood glucose levels are elevated and fasting blood glucose levels are still within normal limits. Blood glucose levels after a meal are elevated.

(3) Stage III: Diabetes is fully expressed with excess release of glucose from the liver and elevated fasting blood glucose levels.

(4) Stage IV: Diabetes complications are seen.

Gestational Diabetes Mellitus (GDM, Diabetes in Pregnancy)

Gestational diabetes affects nearly 9–10% females in pregnancy, especially those over forty years of age, Asians, history of GDM in previous pregnancy or those with a strong family history of diabetes. It is believed that insulin resistance develops in females who are grossly obese. Placental hormones are also implicated in the appearance of GDM. It usually resolves after pregnancy though, it may persist in about 10–12% of females even after pregnancy as diabetes mellitus type II.

Complications of Diabetes

(1) **MACROVASCULAR COMPLICATIONS:** Atherosclerosis (blockages developing in the blood vessels of the heart, brain, kidneys and limbs) which can decrease the blood supply to these organs and cause stroke, heart attacks, unexplained kidney failure, loss of limb or even death.

(2) **MICROVASCULAR COMPLICATIONS:** These occur when the smaller sized blood vessels such as capillaries get inflamed and develop blockages. This leads to permanent damage to some of the sensitive tissues of the body such as the retina in the eye (diabetic retinopathy). This leads to blurring of vision and sometimes even progressive blindness. HEAVY WEIGHT TRAINING IN DIABETIC RETINOPATHY SHOULD NEVER BE ATTEMPTED AS IT CAN LEAD TO RETINAL DETACHMENT AND PERMANENT BLINDNESS. Other microvascular complications include poor wound healing because of lack of blood supply at the tissue and cellular levels.

(3) **DIABETIC NEUROPATHY:** The nerves get damaged because of increased blood and tissue glucose levels. This can lead to tingling numbness in the feet and hands, loss of sensation and

even decrease in the force producing ability of the skeletal muscles.

Diabetes mellitus type II: Through the eyes of a Fitness trainer and Nutritionist

If you deduce logically from the previous chapters and also this chapter about the human body and carbohydrate metabolism, the development of diabetes type II will unfold before you. Moreover, what steps should be taken to ensure its prevention will also become very clear. It will also be obvious why India is becoming the capital of diabetes type II in the world.

In the previous chapter, I had dissected the nutritional value of Indian foods. Our 'Ghar Ka Khana' is loaded with carbohydrates. Human body can contain only 400–500 grams of carbohydrates which is stored in the muscles and liver as glycogen. Our lifestyles have become sedentary. Very few of us indulge in intense workout sessions and resort to simple strolling as a form of exercise. If you perform endurance work, your body burns more of fats and less of carbohydrates. There was a time when access to food was limited and what food did we get before a few thousand years? Animals, fruits and roots. The basic chemistry of the human body has not changed. We still do not have the enzymes to digest plants. Are we really biochemically suited to eat pure vegetarian food? And what do you mean by pure vegetarian food nowadays? Paneer tikka masala, dal makhani and butter naans! Our current pure vegetarian food is carbohydrate and fat loaded. If we actually count the number of times we put food in our mouths during the course of the day, the number should touch 9–10. And that food is usually carbohydrates. Because of our sedentary lifestyles, our carbohydrate stores are usually full even before our next major meal. Carbohydrates are ingested again and insulin is released. But, there is practically no space left in the liver and muscles to store carbohydrates. So, it requires a much higher amount of insulin to bring down the blood sugars. Insulin drives these carbohydrates into the fat cells as there is no other space left. After a few hours, again there is time for the next meal and another insulin spike. Because the insulin is chronically raised, a resistance starts to develop in the tissues towards this insulin. 'FAMILIARITY BREEDS CONTEMPT,' Right? Slowly, a person's metabolism shifts towards insulin resistance and diabetes type II. The fat gain occurring as a result of the above practices contributes to this resistance. Sounds logical? It is. Those researchers who shout about genetics being the cause of diabetes type II should turn towards more simpler and logical explanations. Heredity plays a role in a different way in that we inherit our lifestyles from our parents.

I consider this explanation to be logical, because I started working on my clients in a reverse manner to reverse diabetes type II and I am fairly successful in doing so.

Medical management of Diabetes

GOALS OF MANAGEMENT

- ✧ Achieving good blood sugar level control.
- ✧ Prevention and management of chronic complications of Diabetes.

GUIDELINES FOR DIABETES MANAGEMENT

- ✧ Proper diet.
- ✧ Resistance training (in other words, weight training) which increases skeletal muscle mass and glucose uptake and glycogen synthesis in the muscles without the aid of insulin.
- ✧ If still blood sugars are not controlled, then fine regulation can be achieved by adding certain anti-diabetes drugs and sometimes, insulin.
- ✧ Avoidance of tobacco and alcohol in any form.

Can Diabetes be completely reversed?

Diabetes type I cannot be reversed because the body does not produce enough insulin. But yes, a correct combination of proper diet and weight training program can bring down the blood sugars to normal levels and can prevent long term complications of diabetes.

Diabetes type II is a different ball game. I have given a detailed account on what is the cause of diabetes type II, so if I can reverse these factors, then I can certainly reverse it to a large extent. But, then the person should be ready to change his/her whole lifestyle permanently. The diet should contain very less carbohydrates and that too of the low glycemic index variety. Weight training should be initiated and should be continued till a ripe old age.

Caution: This is a very simplified version of diabetes management and reversal and many of you might be tempted to try it out on your own. It is advisable to refrain from doing it yourself if you do not have the requisite medical and nutritional knowledge as it may lead to complications and can even be fatal. So, take care.

CHAPTER 34

THE TOXICITY OF DETOXIFICATION

This is the latest fad in the market. It seems as if every dietician and naturopathy healer feels that our body is full of toxins and a detoxification diet can clear the body of all its toxins. Many centres have come up offering detox treatment to their clients at an exorbitant expense sometimes amounting to hundreds of thousands of rupees. But, do these practices really work? Let us find out logically.

Toxins enter our body by many routes. Most common is the oral route. Our food what we eat contains many contaminants in the form of pesticides and artificial ingredients. Alcohol ingestion leads to formation of acetaldehyde which is a toxin. Polluted air is inhaled daily by us and many toxic gases enter the body by that route. Some of the addictive substances like marijuana, cocaine, heroin etc. the use of which is very common nowadays can lead to the build-up of toxins in the body. Even our metabolism leads to formation of toxins in the body which are taken care of by the body itself.

How the body detoxifies itself?

Our body has a detoxification centre in the form of liver. Liver is the organ which traps all the toxins in your body and makes them harmless by various chemical reactions. It is a superb organ working twenty four hours a day. The toxins are rendered harmless in the liver and then, released either in the bile to be excreted in faeces or they go to the kidneys where they are filtered out in the urine. Some of the toxins are excreted in sweat in very minute quantities. The liver has a large reserve and most of it has to be non-functional to allow the toxins to build up in the body. Kidney failure can also lead to non-excretion of certain toxic metabolites.

What is detoxification or detox?

Detox is the physiological or medicinal removal of toxic substances from the body, which is mainly carried out by the liver. It can also refer to the withdrawal period after stopping of any addictive substance. Certain poisons if taken accidentally or intentionally can be decontaminated by administration of their antidotes e.g. atropine in organophosphorus poisoning. Chelation therapy can be performed in limited cases. In extreme cases, dialysis can be performed.

Do natural detoxification treatments really work?

Alternative medicine claims to remove 'toxins' from your body through herbal, electrical or electromagnetic treatments. Till now, they have never specified the toxins that they remove. Their claims have no scientific basis. Liver and kidneys are the main organs which detoxify your body. If there is really a build-up of toxins in your body, it means that your liver or kidneys or probably both are not functioning and it is time for you to see a liver specialist or a kidney specialist.

Till now, there is no scientific evidence to believe that there are such toxins which can be removed by natural means. Detox diets though very glamorous and appealing are merely designed to play with your emotions and fears and in reality do not exist. A change over to a healthy lifestyle is the best 'Detox.'

CHAPTER 35

FAT LOSS BLUNDERS

Countless people join the gym daily to cut body fat, but countless people also quit when they do not get the results. If you are one of those, then I am sure you are committing one or many of these blunders.

Most of us spend years trying to get rid of extra body fat with little success. Many fancy drugs are available in the market with tall claims of making you lose the extra flab even if you are gorging on junk food. We spend thousands of rupees on these fancy medicines but, in the end, all we have is the lard still present on our bodies. Many of us go to dieticians who put us on starvation diets which wreck our metabolism. Whenever our motivation is high, we attack our body fat very vigorously, but, when we go out with our families for dinner and our children demand those warm cookies, even we extend our hand for one of those and our motivation for fat loss goes for a six. This stilted progress results in many unfinished New Year's resolutions and scores of dis-satisfied gym clients.

If you have been fighting your body fat for a long time and have not got any success, it is time to introspect whether you are making any of these mistakes mentioned below:

(1) You are eating much more than your maintenance calories. It is an indisputable fact that if your output is less than input, fat has to accumulate.

(2) Much of our food is laden with carbohydrates. There is just not enough protein in our food. Remember, not all calories are equal in quality when they are coming from different food sources. Other than the calories, the food should also contain the right proportions of carbohydrates, fats and proteins.

(3) Many of us feel that as we are hitting the gym, we can burn off any calories. This sometimes results in excessive consumption of empty calories like soft drinks or even alcohol. These excess calories get deposited as fat.

(4) The supermarkets are laden with fat free foods. These foods are loaded with carbohydrates to make them tasty. Remember the previous chapters. Good fats eaten in right quantities are not harmful. Excess carbohydrates are definitely harmful.

(5) We all feel that foods which are considered healthy should be eaten in large quantities without any fear of getting fat. This is not so. Imagine yourself eating oats day and night. They are healthy but, they are one of the richest sources of carbohydrates. Wouldn't it lead to fat gain?

(6) YOU PERFORM VERY LITTLE WEIGHT TRAINING AND TOO MUCH LOW-INTENSITY CARDIO. Just visit any gym. You will find the most obese people on the treadmills. Re-visit the gym after six months. The same clients will still be found on the treadmills. They will be more obese than before. Even if some of them manage to lose weight, it will be more of lean body mass loss rather than fat loss.

(7) Too much stress leads to hormonal imbalances in the body contributing to obesity. Also, many people go on an eating binge during times of stress. Stress can be used as a pretext for consumption of alcohol with disastrous results.

(8) YOU DON'T GET ENOUGH SLEEP. Having a quality sleep 7-8 hours every night leads to significant fat loss. Body recovers during sleep. Stress decreases. You don't consume food during sleep and the body switches to the fat-burning mode. Also, deep sleep induces release of Growth Hormone from the Pituitary gland which has tremendous recuperative potential.

(9) Many people hitting the gym consume proteins on every pretext. You will see people drinking protein shakes throughout the day,

much more than the required quantity of protein to build good quality lean muscle. Excess protein gets converted to fat.

(10) Last but very important reason is that we give in to pressure from family and friends about eating some more at every pretext. These 'THODA THODA' quantities accumulate to form 'JYADA JYADA FAT.'

Nocturnal dietary mistakes

Most people make these common dietary mistakes before bedtime. These mistakes are the result of long-time myths prevalent in the fitness world. It was once thought that eating carbohydrates during bedtime will make you fat. But, many of these myths have been discredited now.

(1) **SKIPPING PROTEINS DURING BEDTIME:** If you have an early dinner, then it is advisable to eat a long digesting protein in the night. Many dairy products contain a protein called 'Casein' which is very slow digesting and hence provides a steady source of protein throughout the night. A casein supplement is available in the market which is a very good source of night time protein.

(2) **NOT EATING CARBOHYDRATES AT NIGHT:** It is the total quantity of carbohydrates eaten throughout the day which is responsible for fat gain or fat loss. If the carbohydrates eaten during dinner fit in your required quantity of carbohydrates, then, you are very unlikely to gain fat. It has been shown in many studies that people who eat major portion of their required carbohydrates during dinner actually lose fat.

(3) **CONSUMING STIMULANTS LATE IN THE DAY:** Stimulants such as coffee or energy drinks which contain caffeine, if taken later in the day can deprive you of quality and quantity sleep that is needed for proper body rest and recovery.

(4) **ALCOHOL CONSUMPTION:** Alcohol, if taken to induce sleep actually hampers sleep. Sleep always comes in cycles in the night; its' stages ranging from light sleep to the deepest sleep. Alcohol keeps the individual in the lighter zones of sleep and

prevents the deep stage and the REM sleep (this is the part of the sleep when a person sees dreams). Growth hormone production happens during the deep zone of sleep, which is responsible for muscle growth and body's reparative processes. It is also a very powerful fat burner. Hence, alcohol is a very poor choice as a sleep inducer. Avoid these fat loss blunders and go for scientific fat loss. I am very sure you will be lean in no time.

CHAPTER 36

INTERMITTENT FASTING (IF): A SURE METHOD TO LOSE FAT AND BUILD MUSCLE

Is breakfast the most important meal of the day? It's time to unlearn this fat loss rule.

In our families and schools and also with all the dieticians and doctors, all of us are hammered with the idea that 'Breakfast is the most important meal of the day. We should breakfast like a king, lunch like a common man and dine like a beggar.' This concept does make sense sometimes as we are consuming most of the calories during the time when we are most active and lesser calories during night when we will be asleep. But, if you think from the body's biochemical point of view, this principle does not hold true.

What happens when you consume large meals during the times when you are most active is that the food what you eat is used as fuel for energy rather than your own fat stores.

When you sleep at night, the body secretes Growth Hormone (GH). This is one of the most potent fat burners known to humans. This ensures that your body is burning its fat stores during sleep. Now, when you wake up, your body secretes stress hormones (cortisol, adrenaline and nor-adrenaline) because the action of waking up and getting out of bed is perceived as stress by the body. Your body is still under the fat-burning influence of GH. Your stress hormones are humming in your blood. This combination plays havoc with your fat stores. If you prolong this fasting state, your body continues to burn its fat stores.

Now, the paradox happens. You consume a very heavy breakfast. This leads to increase in your blood sugar levels and insulin is released in the body in response to this. More than 5 grams of glucose absorbed is enough to release insulin. This insulin shuts off the fat-burning avalanche initiated by GH plus the stress hormones and body switches to burning carbohydrates as fuel.

SO, HOW CAN BREAKFAST BE THE MOST IMPORTANT MEAL OF THE DAY WHEN YOU WANT TO LOSE FAT?

The concept of Intermittent Fasting

Imagine that you do not consume any calories in the morning, not even your good old tea with milk and sugar; in short, you do not consume a single calorie in any form. Your body is under the fat-burning influence of GH released during sleep. Your stress hormones are released in response to your waking up. Your fat stores are being burnt like a furnace. You prolong this fasting state as much as possible. During this time, you will continue to burn fat as fuel. As there is no calorie intake, your blood sugar levels have not risen and no insulin is released. Your body continues to be under the influence of the fat burning effects of GH and the stress hormones. You prolong this fasting state as much as you can, say about 16–18 hours to ensure a good fat burning state. In the absence of insulin, the body becomes very sensitised to it and hence when you consume food, say after an interval of 18 hours, your body is unlikely to store it as fat.

Now, try exercising in the later part of the fasting period just before your first meal of the day. There will be a metabolic mayhem and you will lose pure fat. The anabolic response that will be generated will result in pure muscle gain.

Many people will argue that as you are fasting, your metabolism might drop. This does not hold true in the case of Intermittent Fasting (IF) as your fasting is of a very short duration. When you severely drop your calories over a matter of few days, you will drop your metabolism but, not with a fasting interval of 16–18 hours.

This technique is not a 'diet,' but a specific eating pattern. It is very practical for people who aim to lose fat, but their occupation requires them to travel frequently and who are not able to maintain a very strict diet protocol because of their frequent travelling.

An example of IF

Let's take an arbitrary example of IF. Imagine that you consume your last meal of the day at 8 pm. Try to have your breakfast at 2 pm. Mind you, I am not asking you to skip breakfast, but only to delay it. Take two large meals one at 2 pm and one at 8 pm or three medium sized meals one at 2 pm, one at 5 pm and one at 8 pm. Eat healthy food according to your macronutrient calculations. It would greatly aid in your fat loss if you exercise just before your first meal. Try to fast one entire day in a week. Imagine that you had a heavy dinner on Saturday at 8 pm. Now, fast the entire Sunday and go out with your family at 8 pm and enjoy a lavish feast with them. Sounds great, isn't it!

Lots of people have this notion that they cannot skip breakfast, but it is purely a mind-set. The human body is extremely adaptable. Once you get used to IF, I bet sure you will never want to have breakfast again in your life, as you will radiate a lot of energy during your fasting interval.

DON'T BELIEVE ME? THEN, TRY IT.

CHAPTER 37

EATING DISORDERS

This topic has probably never been covered in any fitness manual or manuscript. But, it has such a profound presence in modern day society that it certainly has earned its place in my book. Eating disorders are actually very common, quite serious and often they are fatal illnesses. Obsessions with food, body weight and shape may signal an eating disorder. These disorders appear usually in teenagers and young adults and are of four kinds:

BINGE EATING DISORDER

The sufferers are those people who lose control over their eating habits. It is usually associated with severe depression in which food is taken as a means of soothing the person or for his/her entertainment. Eating large quantities of food makes the person happy. These people eat even when they are not hungry and they resort to excessive amounts of food which makes them uncomfortably full. They often eat the food in secret to avoid embarrassment and frequently feel guilty about their appetite. These people frequently go for crash starvation diets, but within a very short time, they return back to their binge-eating habits. They are very likely to be grossly obese, along with all the lifestyle diseases like Diabetes type II, Hypertension, Cardiac diseases etc.

NIGHT EATING SYNDROME

In this disorder, the subjects wake up frequently in night and eat food. Usually, they gorge on junk food. These people eat very less food or sometimes, nothing in morning and occasionally, throughout the day. Majority of their food is eaten in night. The productivity of these individuals is often affected as they are unable to maintain healthy sleeping and eating habits. Many of these individuals are grossly obese and are victims of severe stress and depression.

ANOREXIA NERVOSA

These people psychologically see themselves as constantly overweight even when they are grossly underweight. This disorder is mostly found in females who are obsessed about the 'zero figure.' They severely restrict the amount of food they eat and consume only certain foodstuffs. They suffer from an intense fear of gaining weight. They have all sorts of complications associated with starvation namely thinning of bones, muscle weakness and wasting, hair fall and brittleness of nails, severe constipation, infertility, low blood pressure, damage to organs like heart, brain, kidneys, liver etc. severe weakness and feeling tired all the time and even death in extreme cases.

BULIMIA NERVOSA

These people have recurrent and frequent episodes of over-eating followed by a behaviour that compensates for the binge. They indulge in forced vomiting, excessive use of diuretics and laxatives, excessive exercise or a combination of all these behaviours. These people maintain a relatively normal body weight. But, they have complications because of these above mentioned behaviours such as sore throat, tooth enamel damage because of exposure to stomach acids as a result of vomiting, severe acidity, intestinal symptoms like irritation and diarrhoea due to excessive laxative use, severe dehydration and imbalance of minerals in the body which can lead to heart attacks and even paralysis.

How do you manage an eating disorder?

(1) Individual group and family psychotherapy.

(2) Medical care and monitoring.

(3) Nutritional counselling and customised diet plans.

(4) Correct prescription of right exercises.

(5) Medicines such as anti-depressants, anti-psychotics and mood stabilisers.

CHAPTER 38

STRESS AND ILLNESS: ARE YOU STUCK IN HIGH GEAR?

STRESS – the modern disease of mankind!

This is one of my most favourite topics because I deal with the most dreaded complications of stress daily that are 'HEART ATTACKS,' ANGIOPLASTIES and 'BYPASS SURGERIES.'

In this high tech world full of over-achievers, STRESS is bound to occur. We need everything quickly – a big house, a big car, a big business, exotic foreign trips etc. We work long hours for promotions and extra pay packages. We resort to bank loans and then, work like maniacs for meeting the EMIs. Think about it, is it worth if the price is that high?

I ALWAYS TELL PEOPLE THAT YOU CAN EITHER WORK HARD OR WORK SMART. AND SMARTNESS, COMBINED WITH A LITTLE BIT OF TARGETTED HARD WORK CAN WORK WONDERS FOR YOUR CAREER AND LIFE.

Many modern lifestyle diseases are cropping up like Diabetes, High blood pressure, Heart diseases, Gastro-intestinal upsets etc. They all have their links to stress. Many diseases are now known as 'PSYCHO-SOMATIC DISEASES.' Psyche means mind and Soma means body. So, 'Psycho-Somatic disease' means body illness because of mental stress.

YES, IT IS POSSIBLE TO WORRY YOURSELF SICK.

Let us understand what happens when we are stressed. Our body has a hard-wired defence system which induces a 'Fight or Flight response.' This means, whenever our body perceives a threat to its existence, it prepares itself to either fight the situation or run away from the situation. Constant stress, rather than occasional stress, triggers an alarm in the Hypothalamus which is a tiny area at the base of the brain and deals with emotional responses and hormones. The only problem faced is that this alarm always stays on. This activates your adrenal glands situated above your kidneys which leads to a surge of stress hormones such as adrenaline and cortisol. Prolonged stress leads to continuously high levels of these hormones in your body.

What do the stress hormones do?

Adrenaline increases your heart rate, blood pressure and rate of breathing. Cortisol initially increases blood glucose levels and availability of substances for tissue repair. But, very high cortisol levels for a prolonged time can lead to suppression of body's growth processes, reproduction, digestion and immunity.

Medical problems that can be brought on by stress

(1) Coronary heart disease leading to heart attacks and sometimes, death.

(2) Asthma.

(3) Obesity especially around the abdomen and hips (brought on by cortisol excess).

(4) Diabetes mellitus due to unhealthy eating and excessive alcohol consumption because of stress which also predispose the body to obesity.

(5) Headaches due to constant thinking about the problems. It may be in the form of tension headaches or migraine.

(6) Hypertension because of excess adrenaline hormone levels in blood.

(7) Depression and anxiety because of demanding workloads at the workplace and fewer anticipated rewards.

(8) Gastric and intestinal problems like acidity, heart burn, irritable bowel syndrome, ulcers in stomach and intestines etc.

(9)   Early onset of Alzheimer's disease, also called 'senility.'

(10) Accelerated ageing by at least 9–17 years and premature death.

How to manage stress?

(1)   Release tension by physical activity like walking, stair-climbing or indulging in your favourite sport. I hit the gym real hard when I am stressed. More the stress, heavier will be my lifts.

(2)   Healthy Diet.

(3)   Listening to soothing music.

(4)   Talking about the stressful situation with your spouse or your friend who understands.

(5)   Yoga and meditation techniques.

(6)   If possible, remove the stress-producing situation from your life.

(7)   And if nothing helps, consult a medical specialist.

BUT, FOR YOUR OWN SAKE, DON'T LET STRESS
STRESS YOU OUT.

CHAPTER 39

FAD DIETS: AVOID THEM

A Fad diet is a stylish fat loss plan that promises dramatic results. Typically, these diets are unbalanced and not healthy.

A nutrition plan should be designed to meet the energy and metabolic needs of every individual. For example, a person indulging in endurance activities needs much lesser proteins than a bodybuilder. Time should not be wasted in these gimmicks called 'Fad Diets.'

Most of the public is interested in looking for 'quick weight fixes' that are easy to use. They are constantly on the lookout for magic pills or supplements which will make them lose weight without any effort on their part. Most fad diets might result in dramatic weight loss initially, but this weight loss is not fat loss. There is loss of glycogen and water from the body initially, followed by loss of lean body mass, which leads to decrease in metabolic rate. Though some amount of fat is also lost in the process, the fat percentage of the individual may remain the same or actually increase.

Powdered meal replacements usually result in an initial drop in weight which is mostly due to water loss and the gastrointestinal bulk. New gastrointestinal bulk is not formed because these powdered supplements do not contain fibres. Additionally, powdered meal replacements cause diarrhoea which causes significant water loss. Weight loss of this kind is extremely unhealthy and can lead to serious complications.

TARGETTED FAT LOSS ALONG WITH INCREASE IN LEAN BODY MASS IS THE RECOMMENDED METHOD FOR WEIGHT LOSS. The body fat percentage should actually fall because of pure fat loss and not simply weight loss. Increase in lean body mass even with the same amount of fat can also cause decrease in body fat percentage.

As a rule steer clear of those diet plans which does any one of the following:

- ✧ Claims to make you lose weight very quickly.
- ✧ Promises to lower your weight and keep it that way without exercises.
- ✧ Base claims on before-and-after photos.
- ✧ Advertisement from clients and weight loss experts as these people are being paid to advertise.
- ✧ Requires that you spend a lot of money in advance for certain medicines, pre-packaged meals or seminars.

Instead of trying for the 'quick fix' of a fad diet, everyone should make an effort to lose fat through life-long changes in their dietary and exercise habits.

CHAPTER 40

WEIGHT TRAINING: PHYSIOLOGICAL RESPONSES AND ADAPTATIONS

Muscle contractions impose an increased energy demand on the body. Metabolism becomes up-regulated to meet this demand. The entire cardio-vascular system, the lungs, the digestive system as well as the endocrine system (responsible for hormonal production) gear up to tackle this demand. This leads to an overall good impact on the body.

Metabolism

More intense the muscle contraction, more is the ATP used in the contraction. The metabolism fires up to meet the increased ATP demand of the contracting muscles.

Energy demand increases. ATP must provide energy during contractions and also, during recovery from contractions. It should be continuously synthesized during the repetitions in an exercise set. This comes first from your Creatine Phosphate stores in the muscles and later on through glycolysis (splitting of glucose molecules).

How fast the muscle recovers after a set of weight training depends on the ATP and CrP used during the multiple contractions and relaxations of the muscles. As weight training is anaerobic in nature, post-exercise oxygen uptake increases to oxidise the lactic acid produced during the latter part of the set. This increased oxygen uptake may sometimes remain elevated for up to twenty four hours after a weight training session.

The effects on the muscles and the changes happening thereafter have already been explained in the previous chapters.

The Cardio-Vascular System

Increase in muscle mass and body size will lead to more demand of blood supply from the heart. The heart muscle thickens and becomes stronger and leads to more cardiac output. Cardiac Output is the amount of blood pumped by the heart per minute. The heart rate stabilises and does not rise appreciably in response to intense exercise. As compared to that, the heart size actually increases in endurance training such as long distance running.

The Lungs

The work of the lungs increases both during and after exercise and they become more efficient in oxygen intake and carbon dioxide removal.

The Hormones

Acute Stress hormones are released during exercise such as adrenaline. This results in glycolysis and also helps in blood pressure control during exercise. Adrenaline also mobilises fatty acids from the fat stores which can be used as fuel during exercise. Cortisol levels in the blood rise when the weight training session is continued beyond 60 minutes. This leads to mobilisation of amino acids from the muscles and their breakdown to form glucose (gluconeogenesis). This can be offset by taking carbohydrate drinks during a workout session.

Insulin levels decrease during exercise as a result of decreased blood glucose levels. The exercising muscles take up sugar from the blood independent of the action of insulin (this may sound familiar when you read the chapter on diabetes reversal).

Both Testosterone and Growth Hormones are known to increase around 45 minutes into an intense weight training session.

The musculo-skeletal system

Muscle hypertrophy is the direct result of weight training and proper nutrition. There is strengthening of ligaments and tendons as a response to progressively increasing heavy weights. Joints get strengthened because of surrounding muscle hypertrophy and ligament strengthening. Occasionally, you will find cartilage regeneration and remodelling.

One very important end-result as a result of weight training is strengthening of bones. New bone is laid down at the site of stresses applied to the bone due to weight training, especially where the tendons join the bone. You will see in a subsequent chapter how this method can be used to manage and sometimes, even reverse early osteoporosis and osteoarthritis.

CHAPTER 41

WHY WEIGHT TRAINING IS ALWAYS BETTER THAN ENDURANCE TRAINING

I get many long distance runners as clients who want a ripped body like Milkha Singh. I very politely tell them that it might not be possible for them to do so as Milkha Singh was a sprinter and not a marathoner. It is very difficult to build a ripped muscular body if you are running 20 kilometres daily. And we have many fanatics who actually do so. This chapter is for the benefit of all my friends who think that jogging is a good way to get fit.

The evolutionary process

First of all, it should be made clear to everyone that the basic chemical structure of the human body i.e. its biochemistry has not changed much since the time it evolved. The shape might be altered but, the micro-anatomy of the body at the cellular level especially the muscles has not altered. The human body has more of fast-twitch muscle fibres. These are the muscle fibres that have the capacity for explosive activity. There were three basic functions that the human body had to perform before we became sophisticated. But, sophistication has only come at a social level. Otherwise, biochemically we are all the same as our ancestors.

(1) Sprinting after an animal to catch it as food.

(2) Sprinting away from an animal to avoid being its food.

(3) Pushing or lifting a heavy object.

Can you imagine even in olden times that someone is jogging 20–30 miles for catching food or running away from an animal to avoid being its food? Then, if that is the structure of the human body and such is its biochemistry and metabolism, what exactly is the idea behind jogging, running and marathons?

Humans in medieval times were judged by their strength and power and speed and not by their stamina and endurance.

Compare the physique of a marathoner and a sprinter. A sprinter looks like a Greek God with 5-6% body fat and rippling muscles. He/She uses the body for explosive activity and all their fast-twitch muscle fibres are well developed. In comparison, a marathoner has very low amount of lean body mass with more fat percentage.

Why marathoners have a body like theirs'?

Imagine a person running for 20 kilometres almost daily. First of all, no one can maintain a high intensity for that long. So, the running essentially has to be low intensity. Slow twitch muscle fibres develop and fast twitch muscle fibres do not. Slow twitch fibres have the capacity for aerobic metabolism and they do not store an appreciable amount of glycogen in them. Hence, they remain small in size, but at the same time, need a continuous supply of fuel. Now, since very little carbohydrates are stored in them, the body mobilises fatty acids from the fat stores, but that is not all. Exercising more than 60 minutes will lead to a steep rise in the stress hormone cortisol in the body. This cortisol initiates muscle breakdown to provide amino acids for glucose formation (gluconeogenesis), hence the very little lean skeletal muscle mass in them. As more and more fatty acids are being used as fuel, body tries to conserve and store fat so that it can be used during endurance activity. Running daily will lead to a chronically increased cortisol level in the blood. Imagine what can stress hormones do to your body when they are always raised?

Endurance athletes are more exposed to the sun and hence the ageing effect of the ultraviolet rays of the sun on the skin takes its toll. Lots of free toxic radicals are formed in the body as a result of prolonged exercise and sun exposure (the dark side of oxygen). This will naturally make the person more prone to develop diseases caused by increased free radicals. The joints have more wear and tear because of constant impacts, sometimes for hours together, especially those of the ankles and the knees. Many cardiac events are known to happen in marathoners as compared to strength athletes.

Adding insult to injury, a 2004 study published in the Canadian Journal of Applied Physiology showed a remarkable decrease in the testicular size and serum testosterone levels in endurance athletes.

Cardio training for the Cardio-Vascular system

Being a Cardiac Specialist, I fully agree that cardio training is good for the heart, but not the kind of cardio what people do. Simple walking, though it marginally boosts metabolism is not as good an exercise as people and especially doctors think, when fitness is the goal. For old people and people with arthritis, it is a very good exercise, because at least they are doing something. But, when you see young and middle aged people strolling around the parks in the morning and thinking that they have a high level of fitness, then my friends let me assure you that it is not so.

The correct form of cardio training for the young and the middle aged people is HIGH INTENSITY INTERVAL TRAINING. This type of cardio should be performed only for a short duration. It involves a low intensity type of an exercise with sudden short bursts of increased intensity. This gives you a perfect combination of cardio plus high intensity training. Let me give an example. Imagine that you are walking at a brisk pace for two minutes and then, sprinting at top speed for 30 seconds. Complete five rounds of this and believe me, you will be steaming all over, drenched in sweat and your metabolism will shoot through the roof. And when your metabolism is high even at rest, guess what gets burnt as fuel? Fat of course!

CHAPTER 42

ANTHROPOMETRIC CONCEPTS OF WEIGHT TRAINING

What is anthropometry?

Anthropometry is the science that studies the measurements of the size, proportions and composition of the human body. In most of the cases, the measurements are taken directly and combined together to understand the form of the body.

Anthropometric measurement is not what trainers take in the gyms like height, weight, size of the chest, breadth of the shoulders, arms, thighs or calves. Anthropometry refers to the lengths of the individual segments like arms and forearms ratio in upper limbs, ratio of the thigh length and leg length in lower limbs, ponderal index etc.

The knowledge of the basic anthropometric principles is of paramount importance for the correct planning of workouts for a client. Biological individuality means each person will be unique in these measurements. Some people cannot adapt to certain exercises just because of their unique anthropometry, but they benefit from other exercises just because of their unique anthropometry. Interesting, isn't it?

Let me site my own example. For years, I used to perform a lot of Barbell Bench Presses for the development of my chest. My pectoralis major muscle (which is found in front of the chest) never developed. But, my elbow started aching and there was significant soreness in my forearm muscles. My shoulders started hurting. In spite of all this, my pecs looked as if they had never been exercised in life. But, when I applied the principles of anthropometry on myself especially the length of my arms and forearms and the joint angles of the shoulder and the elbow joints, I could deduce that Pect Flyes and Incline Barbell Bench Press would be better exercises for me. I dropped the conventional bench press entirely from my chest workout schedule and performed giant sets of Dumbbell pect flyes and Incline Barbell Bench Press. Within a few workouts, my pecs started growing visibly. This is a classic example how anthropometry can be used for making correct workout schedules.

Not many people benefit from squats. I have many clients who squat really heavy, but their thighs look like those of a ballet dancer. When I figure out their anthropometry, I find that leg presses at a certain angle and foot placement width would be a better alternative to squats for these clients. Lunges would also be a good compliment to leg press. And BOOM! Their legs start growing.

How anthropometric characteristics can be used in fitness and sports?

Many factors contribute to a person's success or effectiveness at a sport or performance at work. You would find that a professional basketball player would be taller than average. Visualise a female gymnast performing floor exercises. If she is very tall, then it would be very cumbersome for her to manipulate her limbs. You would usually find world class female gymnasts smaller in height.

Other measurements affected by training are circumferences of segments (arms, forearms, thighs, and calves), lean body weight, body fat percentage and proportion of various segments. If the various segments of the body are proportionate in size, it looks very pleasing to the eye especially in case of bodybuilding which is quite popular nowadays. If you see the various bodybuilding competitions, you will find the bodybuilder who has developed his various segmental muscles proportionate to each other is the one looking pleasant to the eye. Aesthetic bodybuilding takes into account this aspect of anthropometry.

Anthropometry and movement analysis

Anthropometric characteristics are considered by coaches in selecting athletes for particular sports. The effectiveness of skilled movement patterns are also determined by the mechanical principles used, motor ability (that is ability of the athlete or the individual to perform the movement effectively) and also motivation. I gave you an example of the basketball player and the female gymnast.

Anthropometry and weight training

Anthropometry may determine how effective is your weight training schedule and how much you are prone to getting injured in performance of certain exercises. For example, in performing a deadlift, lifting not only involves the weight of the weighted barbell and the strength of the performer, but other anthropometrically related factors. The height of the performer, the proportion of the lower extremity length to trunk length, the distance the barbell has to travel to reach from the initial position to the final position relative to the lifter's body determine the effectiveness of deadlifts in that particular individual. It also determines how much he/she is prone to injury.

To make squats more effective don't you think a tall person doesn't have to bend much but keep his spine perpendicular to the floor while performing squats, but a short person has to slightly bend forward while going down in deep squats? Don't you think the knowledge of anthropometry helps?

I THINK IT DOES! I AM SCIENTI-FIT!

CHAPTER 43

KINESIOLOGY AND WEIGHT TRAINING

Types of muscles according to their functions

Different muscle groups acting as a team are responsible for movements. Here, I will give an illustration of Biceps curls using a barbell.

(1) **AGONIST:** This is the main muscle which is responsible for the movement. Here, the biceps brachii is the main muscle which curls the arm.

(2) **ANTAGONIST:** The opposite muscle to the biceps is the Triceps brachii found on the back of the arm. This muscle tenses during the biceps curl so that the action of the biceps is carried out in a smooth manner without any jerks. It also lengthens while maintaining the tension.

(3) **SYNERGIST:** They are the muscles which help in the movement. For curling the arm, the brachialis muscle which is found below the biceps and the brachio-radialis muscle which is found on the outer side of the arm also aid in the biceps curl.

(4) **STABILISER:** The deltoids (shoulder muscles) and the Trapezius (muscle of the back found at the back of the shoulder also contract to stabilise the arm during performance of the biceps curl.

(5) **NEUTRALIZER:** Biceps have another function other than curling the arm and that is supination (the movement in which the palm is faced upwards). It would be technically impossible to perform a barbell biceps curl if the forearm is also supinating. Here, the pronator teres muscle which is found on the front of the forearm contracts to neutralise the supination of the forearm. Pronator teres muscle's action is to pronate the forearm that is

moving the wrist in such a way that you can see the back of your hand.

It would sound very surprising to you that so many muscle groups work in synchronous manner to perform a simple task like Barbell Biceps Curl.

Types of muscle contractions

There are basically two main types of muscle contractions based on the tension developed in the muscle:

(1) Isometric contraction in which there is change in tension in the muscle but, there is no change in length.

(2) Isotonic contraction – two subtypes: Concentric and Eccentric. The muscle changes its length with or without change in tension.

Let us see the illustration of Barbell Biceps Curls in light of these two types of contractions.

Imagine yourself curling a heavy barbell. At first, the barbell refuses to move and your biceps becomes tense. The biceps does not shorten, but, the tension in the muscle increases. This is isometric contraction. Holding the barbell midway in the range of motion of a curl is also an example of isometric contraction.

Now, your biceps overcomes the resistance imposed by the weight of the barbell. The tension in the biceps varies only slightly but, it shortens in length. In other words, it contracts. This contraction is also called positive contraction and this phase is known as Concentric Phase.

Now, you are lowering the barbell under control. The biceps lengthens, but stays contracted at the same time. This contraction is also known as negative contraction and this phase is called Eccentric Phase.

Mechanics of muscle growth

We have all heard that micro tears occur in the muscles while lifting and these tears have to be repaired first by the body and then, growth has to happen. Everyone knows and understands this. But, how many trainers and their clients logically follow this?

The muscle contractions can also be divided based on their strengths as follows:

- ✧ Concentric contraction is the weakest contraction.
- ✧ Eccentric contraction is the strongest contraction.
- ✧ Isometric contraction falls in between.

Imagine that you are able to perform a Barbell Biceps Curl only once with a weight of 10 kg. This is the concentric contraction. Now, if I ask you to hold a barbell midway in the range of motion of a curl, you might be able to hold a 15 kg barbell for a few seconds. You might not be able to curl it but, you will certainly be able to hold it. Imagine again that 15 kg is the maximum weight that you can hold. Now, I take away the barbell from your hands and place a 20 kg barbell there and ask you to lower it under full control. You will be able to do so. This is what I mean by the relative strengths of these three types of contractions.

BEYOND FAILURE: THE CONCEPT OF MUSCLE HYPERTROPHY

The concept of muscle failure

You must have heard gym trainers saying about muscle failure countless times. They say that each set of exercise should be carried out till failure; that is, no more repetition of the muscle contraction is possible. Many of their clients also carry out their sets to failure. But, how many of them actually grow? And, if they grow, most of them are hooked to steroids and other juices.

If you follow the advice and principles given in this chapter, I assure you that you can grow your muscles in the shortest possible time. I will not promise you 22" arms, definitely not, but I promise you that whatever is your natural genetic potential for maximal arm circumference (just an example, other body parts need equal or even more attention), you will achieve it in the shortest possible time. You don't need to slog hours in the gym to achieve the body of your dreams; you don't even need to weight train 6 days in a week for your dream physique. All I ask of you is four sessions per week and maybe 30–40 minutes per session. You can utilise your remaining precious time to pursue your vocation or your hobbies. Spend some quality time with your family rather than hitting the gym for 2–3 hours and coming home and dropping dead on the bed.

THERE IS A DIFFERENCE BETWEEN WORKING HARD AND WORKING SMART! YOU SHOULD WORK HARD, BUT SMART!

NEGATIVITY BREEDS GROWTH!

We have seen that there are mainly three different types of muscle contractions; concentric, isometric and eccentric. Let us briefly again shed light on these keeping in our view a simple exercise such as Dumb bell Pect Flyes. In this exercise, you lie down on a bench and hold a dumbbell in each hand. Each wrist should be supinated and your arm should be held perpendicular to your body on its sides. You take a deep breath and bring the dumbbells closer to the midline with the arms held straight ahead. Then, you gradually lower them to the sides.

CONCENTRIC (POSITIVE) CONTRACTION: The motion of bringing the arms from the side of the body to front of the body keeping the arms straight is the concentric phase of Dumbbell Pect Flye.

ISOMETRIC (STATIC) CONTRACTION: You are bringing the arms slowly down to your sides. Midway, you hold the arms steady keeping your chest muscles contracted as long as possible. A burn will start developing in your chest muscles. This is isometric (or static) contraction in which the muscle is under great tension but, there is no movement of the arms.

ECCENTRIC (NEGATIVE) CONTRACTION: The process of bringing the arms to the sides with the dumbbells under full control is the eccentric phase.

The basic universal mistake

The basic universal mistake made by almost every trainer and every client is that the failure of the concentric muscle contraction is misconstrued as the failure of the muscle. People stop their sets short thinking that the muscle has failed. This is where they go wrong. They have merely failed in the concentric contraction. The other two stronger contractions of the muscle, namely the isometric and the eccentric contractions are still a long way to failure.

What exactly is meant by micro tears in the muscles?

MICRO-ANATOMY OF THE CONCENTRIC PHASE

If you remember the chapter on muscles, there are two types of protein filaments in the muscle cells. MYOSIN is a thick filament and ACTIN is a thin filament. Actin and Myosin are arranged in such a way that many actin filaments surround the myosin filaments. When the muscle is relaxed, only the ends of the actin and myosin filaments are overlapping and are united to each other by cross bridges. Rest of the actin filament is free with unfixed cross bridges. When the muscle starts to contract, new cross bridges form between the actin and myosin filaments along the length of the actin fibres and the cross bridges change their shape and shorten by the action of calcium ions which are released by the nerve impulse to the muscle. The actin fibres start sliding over the myosin fibres and new cross bridges are formed which change their shape and shorten and the actin further slides on the myosin. The actin and myosin overlap nearly completely when the muscle is fully contracted. Now, logically thinking, will any micro tears happen in the muscle during the concentric contraction phase because the fibres are coming together and the muscle is getting bunched up? Next to Nil!

MICROANATOMY OF THE ISOMETRIC CONTRACTION

You are holding the weight steady while keeping the muscle partially contracted in the weakest area of the range of motion which is midway in the case of Dumbbell Pect Flye. During this time, the overlap between actin and myosin microfilaments is at a standstill but, new cross bridges are constantly formed and broken down to keep the overlap steady. The muscle is under great tension at this time. There is a rapid turnover of the cross bridges and more and more ATP molecules are used up in the process with a rapid build-up of lactic acid if the isometric phase is maintained for a long time. A few micro tears may happen in the delicate actin and myosin filaments during this phase.

MICROANATOMY OF THE ECCENTRIC CONTRACTION

Now, you are gradually bringing the weight down and your arms to your sides under full control and in a slow and smooth manner. As the movement is very controlled, the muscle has to remain in a contracted state with intact cross bridges between the actin and myosin fibres. But, by the sheer weight of the dumbbells as the arms are being lowered to the sides and as the cross bridges are intact, small micro tears start to form in the actin and myosin filaments in between the cross bridges. It is the negative phase which leads to the maximum micro tears in the muscle fibres.

Negativity breeds growth in body building

We have seen in the previous chapter that the eccentric contraction is the strongest, the concentric contraction is the weakest and the isometric contraction is in between. You have also seen the microanatomy of each phase and how the micro tears happen in the muscle fibres. This is the concept behind 'ECCENTRIC TRAINING.'

Even I agree that muscle failure leads to muscle growth. But, it is not only the concentric failure that matters. Even if the muscle fails to lift the weight, it still has more than enough power to manage even heavier weights in the isometric contraction and still heavier weights in the eccentric contraction. Now, if you can induce an eccentric failure in the first or second set itself, you don't have to continue hitting set after set of an exercise in the gym in order to gain muscle size. This is what I mean by WORKING HARD, BUT SMART.

Let us take an arbitrary eccentric set. Imagine that you can perform Dumbbell Pect Flyes with 15 kg dumbbells in each hand. After a thorough warm up of the exercising body part (in this case, the chest), I ask you to hold a 25 kg dumbbell in each hand. I fully assist you in the positive phase, but, I ask you to lower the weight very slowly to your sides with static contractions in between the range of motion. There has to be a very deep stretch at the lowermost end of the range of motion. This stretch is to be held as long as possible. Again, in the next repetition, I assist you completely in lifting the weight; but, again you lower the weight on your own very slowly under full control with static contraction in the mid-range of motion as long as possible. Again, when you are not able to hold anymore, you lower the weight extremely slowly with a full stretch at the end which is to be held for as long as possible. Repeat this till the eccentric contraction has failed. I bet after such a single set of Dumbbell Pect Flyes, your chest will not be in a position to perform even one set of light weights (you can forget the heavy ones).

THIS IS MUSCLE FAILURE. AND NEGATIVE TRAINING INDUCES THE MAXIMUM NUMBER OF MICRO TEARS IN YOUR MUSCLE, HUNDREDS OF TIMES MORE THAN FOLLOWING JUST CONCENTRIC TRAINING WHICH MOST OF US DO IN THE GYM.

Now, as the isometric and the eccentric contractions have to be taken into account in each repetition, a single set takes about 3 minutes to be completed. Now, imagine yourself hitting a set of Incline Barbell Bench Press immediately after a 'negative' set of Dumbbell Pect Flye. I bet you will achieve failure within 5–6 repetitions. Immediately perform a third set of Cable Cross overs with light to moderate resistance and you have achieved a superb 'pump.' And believe me, your chest muscles will be smarting for more than a week.

WORK HARD, BUT SMART!

More is never better in logical and smart bodybuilding

All of us have been hammered with the idea that more is always better. We try to correlate this with bodybuilding also. We surf the internet and download the workout of our favourite bodybuilder, our idol and follow the workout religiously. Body parts are hit twice or sometimes even thrice in a week. But, what all of us fail to take notice is that your idol body builder is on high doses of Anabolic Chemicals (steroids, peptides and many others). When these compounds are injected in the body, muscle recovery is faster and hence, they can afford to hit various body parts multiple times per week. And even if we poor mortals perform these workouts, we only concentrate on the concentric phase of the training. And then, we crib that our body is not changing and we give up.

REST: The most important factor in natural bodybuilding

Imagine and visualise yourself again hitting that one set of Dumbbell Pect Flye followed immediately by a single set of Incline Barbell Bench

Press followed by a single set of Cable Crossovers. Your 'Pecs' are on fire. Micro tears have extensively formed in your muscles. Give them time to heal before beginning the next chest workout. The soreness will go within a few days but, the tenderness may last for a week or sometimes more. Tenderness means the pain that is felt when you touch a particular body part. Make sure your tenderness goes away completely before you hit the body part again. Eat a proper diet based on your requirements and goals and take a sound sleep. I bet with just one single giant set like this, your sleep will be very sound for the rest of the week. The micro tears which have developed as a result of your eccentric training should heal first for the muscle to regain its former architecture. The next phase that comes is muscle growth. All this takes time; certainly much more than the 2–3 days which all of us have imbibed our minds with. With this eccentric training, your tenderness will last more than a week. Once again, do not go for the workout of that body part which is still tender. Give it time to grow. Eat a good nutritious meal with high protein and some amounts of good fats. And see the muscles grow.

The pump

All of us have heard about 'THE PUMP.' The exercising muscle swells after a workout. This is the pump. Pump is nothing but the accumulation of tissue fluids and blood in the exercising body part. Pump is not the same as muscle growth. Pump merely makes sure that the exercising muscles are getting enough nutrients and blood at the time of exercising and soon thereafter. It usually subsides within a few hours.

A short and not-so-sweet workout

By following these principles, you can make your workout short and, of course, not so sweet. You will witness muscle growth like never before. I once again state that I do not promise you a herculean body when you follow these techniques; that is purely genetics; but, I assure you that whatever will be your genetic potential, these techniques will make you realise it fully.

Universality of bodybuilding principles

The more I think about bodybuilding from the point of view of a doctor (who has an intimate knowledge about the microanatomy, physiology and biochemistry of the human body), a trainer and a nutritionist, the more flaws I find in the 'theories' of the so-called authorities of bodybuilding.

One thing is certain that exercise science is an extension of medical science. How a body functions is same for almost all individuals. Otherwise how can medicines be developed? For example, Paracetamol will bring down the fever in almost all individuals. It can never happen that Paracetamol will increase the fever. There are specific medicines developed for specific effects on the human body. A medicine that decreases the blood pressure will have the same effect in all individuals. It can never have the reverse effect. Digestion of food stuffs, the different enzymes necessary for assimilation of various macronutrients in the body or the micro anatomical structure of the muscle remains the same. The mechanism of muscle contraction is the same in all the persons.

The more I study the form, mechanics and functions of the human body, the more convinced I am that all human beings have the same structure and function. Minor variations are there in form of shape of muscles, their length, and the ratio of segments of the body or the joint angles. But, the microstructure of the muscles, tendons, bones and ligaments are the same. So, if 20 or 200 or even 2000 people want to develop their muscles, how can the basic workout be different for each of them?

Flaws in the concepts of the 'Pundits of bodybuilding'

(1) All experts say that each individual is different and hence, the workouts also should be different. If so, then why everyone advocates that there should be 4–5 different exercises for each body part and each exercise should be having 4–5 sets of 8–12 repetitions each? On one hand, they advocate individuality and on the other hand, there are same number of sets and repetitions prescribed for everyone. Then, where is the individuality?

(2) There is a lot of confusion regarding the words 'Intensity' and 'Volume.' Let me make these terms clear once again. Intensity refers to the intensity of muscle contractions. More intense the contraction, more is the intensity. More is the intensity, more is the fatigue. And when the muscle fibres are fatigued as a result of high intensity, they stay fatigued for a long time. In such a scenario, it is technically impossible for anyone to perform more sets (volume). So, logically, Intensity and Volume can never.......... never............never go together. If someone tells me that they lift really heavy and their workouts last long, I take it that they are kidding!

(3) When the goal is pure muscle building, one thing has to be clearly understood by all the fitness trainers and experts: MUSCLES RESPOND TO PROGRESSIVE OVERLOAD MORE THAN VARIATIONS.

More number of sets means more time spent in the gym. Unless the workout is highly intense, there will not be a surge of anabolic hormones like Growth Hormone and Testosterone to the quantity required in building muscle. On the contrary, the stress hormones will increase which will eat away your muscles. That is why thousands of people give up gymming because they do not have a real body to show for the countless hours and the thousands of bucks spent in the name of personal training and supplements. Fitness industry forces you to eat more and more supplements which ultimately burns a big hole in your pocket rather than burning the extra flab on your waist. It is established that eating more than the required amount of protein will also lead to excess fat gain. But, there is so much peer pressure that people don't mind guzzling down a protein shake at every opportunity.

THE PATH OF LOGICAL THINKING IS VERY LONELY!

CHAPTER 45

HIGH INTENSITY TRAINING PROTOCOLS

The misconception of 'Intensity'

Ask any average gym goer or ask any trainer for that matter about an intense workout. I bet sure most of them will say that intensity means a properly focussed workout or a workout performed rapidly with very little rest in between sets or exercises or supersets or giant sets and so on. But, here I would once and for all like to make a bold and final statement: THIS IS NOT CALLED AN INTENSE WORKOUT.

INTENSITY REFERS TO THE INTENSITY OF MUSCLE CONTRACTION AND NOTHING ELSE.

In the previous chapter, I have demonstrated a chest workout for you, how with a single negative set, we could create a mayhem of micro tears in the Pectoralis muscle of the chest. This chapter will deal on how intense you can make your workout, even beyond the eccentric failure of the muscle. There are hundreds of different techniques found in the literature but, I will enumerate what I found to be most beneficial in my bodybuilding clients.

Giant sets

Giant sets means performing two or three sets of the same body part one after the other with no rest in between. Imagine that you have performed a set of Dumbbell Pect Flyes to failure by following the eccentric technique. Immediately, go for a heavy set of Incline Barbell Bench Press. As your chest muscles are nearly exhausted, you might want to take the help of a trainer or a partner. Incline Bench Press will hit your Pectoralis muscle at a different angle. You will now have

3D micro tears of your Pectoralis. Perform a heavy set with all the three phases of the muscle contraction taken to failure, namely the concentric, isometric and the eccentric phase. This one set is enough to show you stars in the daytime. Immediately following this, go for a single set of cable crossovers with a relatively lighter weight. This finishes a giant set. With these three sets, you can conclude your chest workout in less than 10 minutes and create such an anatomic and metabolic environment locally in the muscle that all you now need is proper nutrition and adequate rest for the muscle to recover. AND, IT WILL DEFINITELY GROW, IT HAS TO!

Giant sets can be performed for various body parts e.g. T-bar rows for the back immediately followed by Wide grip Lat pulldowns for the back. It saves time and as the muscle is already partially failed with the first set, very few repetitions are needed in the second set to carry the muscle to complete failure.

Giant sets, if done properly, can create a very favourable nidus for muscle growth. They certainly save a lot of time and are a perfect example of working smart, unless you are a masochist who likes to torture yourself by continuing to dole out sub-standard sets one after the other.

FORCED REPS

You are hitting a particular exercise and have achieved failure on the concentric contractions of the muscle. Your partner will assist you to finish a few more repetitions of the exercise. I feel that this is the most common scenario we see in the gym and is of little importance in rapid muscle growth.

FORCED NEGATIVE REPS

I feel this is a better technique to build muscle than simple forced reps. During the negative phase, your partner applies pressure so that the negative phase becomes harder for you. This is an advanced form of eccentric training and should be done by advanced weight trainers only.

DROP SETS

Now, this is a good technique for the intermediate trainer. After the muscle is completely exhausted even in the eccentric phase, the weight that is handled is quickly dropped to a lower weight and the set is continued. When the failure is reached again, the weight is further decreased and the set is continued. This technique assures that the last bit of muscle fibre is completely exhausted and no more repetition of that set or that body part for that matter, is possible.

PRE-EXHAUSTION PRINCIPLE

When you perform a compound exercise for a particular muscle group, you will find that the synergist muscles fail much before the main muscle. Hence, the main agonist muscle does not have the stimulus nor the nidus to grow. A classic example is the Bench Press. There are three major muscles involved in performing a Bench Press. They are the Pectoralis Major muscle situated on the front of the chest, the anterior head of the deltoid muscle situated in the front part of the shoulder and the triceps muscle situated at the back of the arm. It is the triceps muscle which always fails first, hence the particular set of the Bench Press is stopped much before the Pectoralis gets exhausted. Lot of people resort to isolation movements in the later part of the workout such as Pec Decks or machine flyes or cable flyes to exhaust the pectoralis muscle. In the pre-exhaustion technique, the isolation movement is done first such as the Pec Deck machine for isolated contraction of the Pectoralis Major muscle. This is immediately followed by a set of heavy Bench Press taken to failure using any of the techniques mentioned above. This method gives an excellent muscle breakdown and a good stimulus for growth.

SUPERSETS

A superset is a combination of two sets performed for opposite muscle groups e.g one set of Barbell Curl for the biceps followed immediately by one set of Triceps push downs. Rest is taken after the second set. In this technique, you can do more work in a short time. Initially, you might not be able to go heavy, but as your system gets used to this, you will gradually be able to take more weights and build muscle. Personally, whatever the literature says, I believe supersets are more useful for cutting rather than bulking that is when you want to lose fat while preserving your existing muscle mass.

REST PAUSE TECHNIQUE

You start with a set that is very heavy (90% of your 1 rep max. I RM means the weight that you can lift for a particular exercise with proper form for only one repetition). Perform 5-8 reps. When the muscle is fatigued, take a rest for a few seconds and then have a go at it again. After the muscle has failed, decrease the weight incrementally and try to dish out as many repetitions as possible. This method is very similar to drop sets, except here you take a pause of about 10–15 seconds in between.

WORK HARD, BUT SMART!

CHAPTER 46

GAINS FOR THE HARDGAINER

Ectomorphs are the men and women who are genetically prone to remain skinny. In spite of eating all kinds of food in whatever quantity, they are unable to gain any weight because of an extremely fast metabolism compared to an average person. They generally tend to be poor eaters though there are abundant examples of the opposite types who eat whatever is in sight and still remain skinny.

These people have a small bony structure i.e. narrow shoulders, flat chest, narrow waist and hips, small wrists and ankles. They are sometimes on the lankier side with tall height, long and gangly limbs and longer than average muscle belly length.

Many people feel that ectomorphs are the 'blessed type' and they can eat any kind of food including junk food and still remain slim. But, sadly that is not true. They have a poor musculature and when they start gaining fat, they become skinny-fat. Now, who would want that kind of a body?

This chapter is not about how ectomorphs should gain weight, but it is about how ectomorphs can gain lean body weight.

How to make a hard gainer gain lean body weight

Muscles grow through three approaches: progressive overload, proper nutrition and an anabolic environment. Performing High Intensity Training for about 30 minutes will lead to a surge in Growth Hormone and Testosterone levels which will create a proper anabolic environment for growth. Now, bearing the above points in mind, let us put a hard gainer on a gaining mode.

(1) Limit weight training to about 30–40 minutes.

(2) Perform more of compound exercises and less of isolation exercises so that, proper Growth Hormone and Testosterone secretion is initiated.

(3) High Intensity Training.

(4) Limit cardio to about 15 minutes two to three times a week.

(5) Eat more calories and higher proteins than normal. Hard gainers can also indulge in frequent cheat meals and get away with them because of their fast metabolism. But, try to keep the diet as clean as possible. They should be eating multiple meals in a day preferably every 2–3 hours.

(6) Proper rest and recovery is a must for them.

REMEMBER ONE GOLDEN RULE: THERE CANNOT BE A GENERAL RULE FOR EVERYONE, NOR THE TIMING OF RESULTS!

CHAPTER 47

THE ART OF FEMALE BODY-SCULPTING

We all must have seen numerous articles on the internet and fitness magazines regarding building your dream physique, but if you look closely at the exercise protocols, they are all for males. The same workouts might not be applicable for females. Why does she need to grind through set after set of different variations of exercises? Why does she need the separation of all the three heads of the deltoid muscle (the shoulder) or delineation of both the heads of her biceps? Hilarious, isn't it? Let us see what should be the correct prescription of exercises for a female.

Most females desire a curvaceous physique with well-toned arms and legs. They want a nice butt that fits the jeans. Think about an ideal female body. She should have around 18–20% of body fat, well-toned thighs, calves, buttocks and back, firm and rounded arms and a flat belly. Along with these physical attributes, there is one disregarded aspect of female body sculpting and that is flexibility.

Reducing body fat percentage is mainly a function of diet, but what's the best way to build a firm body mentioned above? Weight training, of course! I can already see many females disagreeing with me that lifting heavy weights will make them look like bulky bodybuilders, but that statement is far from the truth. The hormone that directly regulates muscle growth is TESTOSTERONE and a female's testosterone level is only 5–10% that of a male. Hence, unless a female is having gross hormonal imbalances or is on high doses of steroids, she can never develop those hulking muscles.

Benefits of building muscle in a female

(1) Your chances of developing diabetes, hypertension and cancer are greatly reduced.

(2) Your bones become stronger. After menopause, many females suffer from osteoporosis (thinning of bones because of loss of calcium). This can be prevented or greatly delayed.

(3) Your metabolism speeds up, thus helping you to stay lean.

(4) Your life expectancy increases.

(5) Your immunity increases.

(6) And what about the feminine physique? Strong firm muscles will give the female the curves that she desires.

(7) And a strong well-developed body helps you age gracefully.

Structuring of a female workout plan

Both weight training and cardio are equally important in a female. Her workout should include the following components in the order given below:

(1) Activation movement for speed and agility. Go for at least 20 repetitions for proper warm-up and to get the blood flowing.

  ✧ Box jumps on leg day.

  ✧ Chest pass with medicinal ball on Chest day.

  ✧ Kettlebell swings (preferably with one arm) on Back day.

  ✧ Standing overhead throw with medicinal ball on Shoulder day.

(2) Compound movements for muscle strength. Go heavy 5 sets X 5 repetitions.

  ✧ Squats.

  ✧ Deadlifts.

  ✧ Lunges.

  ✧ Pull-ups.

  ✧ Dips.

  ✧ Bench Press.

  ✧ Push-ups.

  ✧ Push press.

(3) Accessory/isolation lifts. Include at least 3 per session and go for 3 sets X 8–12 repetitions each.

- ✧ Biceps curls.
- ✧ Triceps extensions.
- ✧ Calf raise.
- ✧ Leg curls.
- ✧ Leg extensions.

Progression is the key. Keep increasing the weights in every session or decrease the rest periods between sets. You can't do the same movements with the same weights and expect new results.

(4) Cardio: High intensity interval training should be done after the weight training for 20 minutes to promote fat loss.

Low intensity cardio: You can jump on your favourite elliptical cross trainer for 30 minutes once in a week to build up your stamina. Just make sure you don't do it on our weight training days.

(5) Stretching movements for flexibility.

AN IDEAL WORKOUT SCHEDULE SHOULD LOOK LIKE THIS:

Monday: Back and Biceps.

Tuesday: Chest and Triceps.

Wednesday: Low intensity cardio.

Thursday: Shoulders and Abdomen.

Friday: Legs and Calves.

Saturday: HIIT and Core training.

Sunday: Rest day.

So, ladies, it is high time that you put down those pink play-weights and get sexy by lifting heavy like the guys. Eat clean and sculpt your dream body.

CHAPTER 48

RIGHT TO BE FIT: FITNESS IN SOME MEDICAL CONDITIONS

I do not think any client should be denied the right to fitness just because he/she is suffering from some medical condition. The conditions what I am going to enumerate are all lifestyle ailments and if lifestyle can be modified, then I am sure most of these conditions can be drastically reduced in severity or even be managed without medications. Though being a medical specialist makes me feel that drug therapy should be the cornerstone of more severe cases, the less severe ones could be dealt with exercises and correct diet plans so that the need for drugs can be greatly reduced or completely abolished.

Hypertension

When the heart pumps i.e. when it squeezes blood through the arteries, the pressure that is generated is called the 'Systolic blood pressure.' During the relaxation phase of the heart, that is when the heart relaxes in between two squeezes, the pressure generated is known as the 'Diastolic blood pressure.' The arteries are elastic in nature. When they recoil against the pressure of the blood flow, diastolic blood pressure is generated. If the blood pressure of a person is let's say 150/90 mm Hg, the higher value that is 150 is the systolic blood pressure and the lower value that is 90 is the diastolic blood pressure.

Hypertension is a chronic medical condition in which the pressure of the blood flow in the arteries is higher than normal. The heart has to work harder to circulate the blood through its network of blood vessels. It is a risk factor for diseases like cardiovascular episodes, heart attacks, stroke etc.

TYPES OF HYPERTENSION

(1) Primary hypertension which is present in more than 95% of patients. No cause is determined for this yet, but, newer researches have labelled it as a lifestyle ailment.

(2) Secondary hypertension is present in less than 5% of the patients. There are specific causes attributed to this type such as narrowing of the artery supplying the kidney, tumours of the adrenal gland etc.

Various factors such as age, sex, height, ethnicity, genetics etc. influence the BP of an individual. It can also vary with exercise, emotions, sleep, digestion and time of day (circadian rhythm). In the elderly, the BP tends to be slightly higher than normal range (130–120/80–70 mm Hg) and the cause is said to be reduced elasticity of the arteries in old age.

STAGES OF HYPERTENSION

Optimal: <120/80 mm Hg.

Pre-hypertension stage: 120–139/80–89 mm Hg.

Stage I hypertension: 140–159/90–99 mm Hg.

Stage II hypertension: >160/100 mm Hg.

The risk of cardiovascular diseases and stroke progressively increases starting from the pre-hypertension stage.

WHAT SHOULD BE THE BP GOALS THEN?

According to the 7th guidelines given by the Joint National Committee, US, the BP goals should be as follows:

- ◈ Less than 140/90 mm Hg in patients with uncomplicated hypertension.

- ◈ Less than 130/85 mm Hg in diabetes and those with kidney disease and if no protein is present in the urine.

- ◈ Less than 125/75 mm Hg in patients with kidney disease and presence of protein in the urine.

MANAGEMENT OF HYPERTENSION

Various methods have been advocated such as:

- ✧ Lifestyle changes and dietary modifications.
- ✧ Exercise programs.
- ✧ Drugs.
- ✧ Rarely, surgery/catheter treatment of any identifiable cause of hypertension such as tumour of the adrenal gland, narrowing of the artery supplying the kidney etc.

IS HYPERTENSION REVERSIBLE?

Many cases of mild to moderate primary hypertension are reversible by

- ✧ Lifestyle modification.
- ✧ Correct nutritional modifications.
- ✧ Modified exercise techniques.
- ✧ Cessation of smoking, alcohol etc.
- ✧ Stress relieving therapies.

Caution is advised against self-manipulating your lifestyle without the guidance of an expert because patients have been known to lose lives when the BP fluctuates dangerously.

Hypothyroid as a lifestyle disease

I have come across hundreds of patients who are supposed to be hypothyroid and are on thyroid hormone replacement therapy. There seems to be a sudden hypothyroidism epidemic in India. But, what is the truth? Let us review the anatomy, physiology and biochemistry of the thyroid gland and how is it relevant in finding out the truth.

Thyroid is a dumbbell shaped gland situated in the neck in front of the windpipe. This gland produces thyroid hormones which influence practically every cell in your body. The thyroid gland regulates the body's metabolism and also other aspects like maturation, energy levels, heart rate and brain function.

CAUSES OF HYPOTHYROIDISM

(1) Iodine deficiency: Iodine is a mineral needed by the body in trace quantities for formation of thyroid hormones. Deficiency of this is the commonest cause of hypothyroidism. This article will purely focus on iodine deficiency and how it is very often mis-diagnosed as hypothyroidism.

(2) Hashimoto's disease: In this disease, the body's immune system attacks its own thyroid gland.

(3) Other rare causes are radiation, certain food stuffs, surgery on the thyroid gland etc.

MISDIAGNOSIS OF HYPOTHYROIDISM

Iodine is a mineral which is required in trace amounts by the human body for the formation of thyroid hormones. The richest sources are seafood, plants found near the sea shores, milk, eggs, turkey, navy beans etc. Nowadays, we are getting iodine fortified salts. Whenever there is iodine deficiency in the body, the iodine trapping mechanism in the thyroid gland becomes more efficient in conserving iodine. The thyroid gland tries to increase the formation of T3 hormone from T4 hormone (both these hormones are formed in the thyroid gland; T3 is the more active form). If you remember, there is a negative feedback loop in the body when it comes to thyroid hormone production. Thyroid gland is a burner and pituitary gland is a thermostat. When the burner is running low, the thermostat switches on. When there is iodine deficiency, the TSH levels rise. I get many clients who are diagnosed with hypothyroidism. When you see their reports, their T3 and T4 levels are normal or T3 is slightly raised as mentioned above. The TSH levels are elevated. These reports indicate iodine deficiency and not hypothyroidism, and patients are wrongly prescribed thyroid hormone replacement therapy and not iodine supplementation. In other words, you are stifling the burner and switching off the thermostat.

I do not really think there is such a surge of hypothyroid cases as people think, but there is definitely a higher incidence of iodine deficiency which can be completely reversed by modifying your diet.

LIFESTYLE MODIFICATIONS TO MANAGE THESE CASES OF IODINE DEFICIENCY

(1) Eating food rich in iodine such as mentioned above.

(2) There are certain food items such as cabbage, cauliflower, broccoli and soya beans which are known to suppress thyroid hormone production and cause goitre (swelling of the thyroid gland). Their use should be decreased.

(3) Increase intake of complex carbohydrates. They are known to stabilise your thyroid hormones in the blood.

(4) Drink a lot of water.

(5) Sleep at least 7–9 hours daily.

(6) Strength training with right amounts of cardio will boost your metabolism.

(7) Decrease stress by meditation and other relaxing techniques.

Polycystic ovarian disease (PCOD)

I have seen a lot of fitness gurus harping about PCOD reversal through diet and exercise. My views are slightly reserved in this condition.

PCOD is a set of symptoms due to elevated androgens (male sex hormones) in females. Signs and symptoms include irregular or no menstrual periods, excess body and facial hair, acne, pelvic pain and infertility (difficulty in conceiving).

PCOD is due to a combination of genetic and environmental factors. The risk factors are obesity, sedentary lifestyle and a strong family history. There are three main findings in PCOD: no ovulation, high male hormones and multiple cysts present in the ovaries. The root cause of PCOD is abnormal hormonal levels, which is genetic though obesity increases the severity of PCOD. High levels of fatty tissue in the body of a PCOD female increases conversion of the already increased male hormones to oestrogen, which decreases the pituitary gland function in the female. Pituitary gland is the main gland in the body which regulates the blood levels of most hormones of the body. FSH is a hormone produced by the pituitary and is responsible for formation of oestrogen and maturation of the ovarian follicles and egg production in the female. High levels of androgens and oestrogen in the female suppress FSH production by the pituitary and hence, these females do not ovulate.

Obesity in PCOD patients can be the cause of insulin resistance and type II diabetes seen in many of these patients.

There are many diseases of the pituitary, thyroid and adrenal glands which can produce symptoms similar to PCOD. These other conditions should be categorically investigated and ruled out by a doctor before the female is labelled as having PCOD.

My take on the management of PCOD is that there is a genetic cause behind it. It cannot be completely reversed regardless of whatever claims people make. But, you can certainly decrease the symptoms of PCOD by these measures:

(1) Weight reduction: Not all PCOD patients are obese. But, whenever obesity is present, diet and exercise play a major role. These patients benefit from a low carbohydrate diet and vitamin D supplementation. Though successful weight reduction restores ovulation in many of these females, they find it very difficult to sustain their weight loss for a long time. Their lifestyle has to be changed completely. Exercises have to be continued as long as possible along with dietary modifications. Weight reduction can improve insulin sensitivity and can sometimes even reverse diabetes type II in these cases.

(2) Medications include oral contraceptive pills to regularise periods and Metformin which sometimes stabilises ovarian function. Clomiphene citrate can sometimes induce ovulation in these patients. Drugs are known to reduce hirsutism (increased facial hair like a male).

DRUG TREATMENTS DO NOT WORK IN ALL PATIENTS.

(3) Occasionally, surgery helps.

The final conclusion is that treatment of PCOD includes attack on all fronts with the right hormonal assessment and continuous monitoring, diet, exercises and medications.

Yes, patients with PCOD can lead fruitful lives.

Osteoporosis: can it be reversed?

During life, there is constant remodelling of the bone. Old bone is destroyed and new bone is formed. The formation of new bone is maximum amongst pre-pubertal and pubertal age groups which causes growth. This gets balanced during adult life. During old age, formation of new bone slows down and destruction of old bone continues at the same rate. Because of this, the bone becomes fragile. Often, the first indication of osteoporosis is fracture.

Osteoporosis can be diagnosed by tests known as BONE MINERAL DENSITY (BMD) and BONE MINERAL CONTENT (BMC). These tests often show that approximately 25% bone loss is there when osteoporosis happens.

80% of osteoporosis patients are females. Other factors are sedentary lifestyle, disordered eating, amenorrhoea, nutritional deficiencies etc. As you can see, most of these factors can be modified.

PREVENTION must take place during each stage of the life cycle. Achieving peak bone mass during childhood, adolescence and early adulthood, maintaining bone mass through middle age and minimising bone loss during old age are the cornerstones of prevention.

Optimizing BMD and BMC in early life leads to reduction in risk of osteoporosis. Weight bearing and strengthening exercises that load the skeleton via muscular contractions (as in weight training) are powerful contributors to maximising peak bone mass.

MANAGEMENT OF OSTEOPOROSIS

Osteoporosis usually involves the vertebrae, the thigh bone at its attachment with the hip (known as Femur neck) and the wrist. First, we have to identify the sites where osteoporosis has set in by performing a bone scan.

Weight training can increase bone density by providing periodic increases greater than the habitual loads applied to bone. Usually, the minimal essential strain (the minimum weight that initiates new bone formation) is theorised to be the force per unit area approximately equal to 10% of the force needed to fracture that particular bone. This means safe weight training if applied correctly can initiate new bone formation at the osteoporotic site within 8–12 weeks of beginning weight training. The weights that are used will vary amongst individuals based on history of exercises done in past and current type and level of activity. BMD usually increases within six months of following these exercises.

The bones of the vertebrae (spine) usually respond better to weight training than the bones of the limbs.

SPECIAL RECOMMENDATIONS FOR WEIGHT TRAINING IN OSTEOPOROSIS

Before starting weight training, a proper medical screening and evaluation, including medical history and a current health status should be done. BMD and a bone scan should be done to obtain information about the specific bone regions at risk of fracture, and to monitor changes in bone over time. Assessment of exercise history, current exercise participation, joint stability, flexibility and strength should also be done.

Weight training to maximise bone health should always be performed for a minimum period of one year and preferably throughout the life of the individual. The most beneficial exercises for bones use muscles that originate or insert at the sites of osteoporosis in the bone.

EXERCISES TARGETTING THE HIP ROTATOR MUSCLES AND ADDUCTORS will contribute significantly to increase BMD of the femoral neck.

Leg extensions and Leg flexions including Leg presses and Squats will increase new bone formation in the upper part of thigh bone (femur).

FOR INCREASING BMD OF THE WRIST, exercises that use brachioradialis and pronator quadratus muscles such as arm curls with forearm rotations, wrist curls and reverse wrist curls should be done.

FOR OSTEOPOROSIS OF THE SPINE, bent knee deadlifts and cleans that engage both the superficial and deep back and spinal muscles, lat pull downs and back and hip extension exercises should be done.

Weight training should be done at the proper intensity, volume of bone loading (number of exercises, sets and repetitions) and be of sufficient duration to increase the BMD.

Yes, Osteoporosis can be prevented and even treated in many cases. But, please do not attempt the above mentioned regimens yourself without expert supervision.

CHAPTER 49

FITNESS DURING AND POST PREGNANCY

There is a lot of misconception about exercises in pregnancy. Many females think that during pregnancy, they should take proper rest and eat a lot of food. The result is rapid weight gain which gets compounded even after delivery and then, the female accepts the obesity as her way of life. But, nowadays, females have at last woken up to the fact that it is always better to live a fit life in order to prevent all the lifestyle ailments what they might acquire in middle age. Exercises help in an uncomplicated pregnancy and a healthy baby. This chapter is dedicated to all the females who think like that. It will remove many misunderstandings about fitness during pregnancy and after delivery.

Exercise in Pregnancy

The more active and fit you are during pregnancy, the more easier it will be for you to adapt to your changing shape and weight gain during pregnancy. It will also help you to have an easier labour or a caesarean section and to get back in shape very fast post-pregnancy.

Exercises that you might be doing before you got pregnant (except very heavy weight lifting exercises) such as light sports, running, yoga, dancing or even walking can be continued during pregnancy if it is comfortable for you. One important thing to remember is that you should not exhaust yourself. During exercises, you should be able to speak comfortably. If you are feeling breathless while exercising, then it shows that the exercise is too intense for you and you should slow down. Remember that during pregnancy, the exercises need not be too strenuous to be beneficial.

EXERCISE TIPS DURING PREGNANCY

✧ Always warm up before the exercises.

✧ Try to perform the exercises on a daily basis. If you can't exercise, even daily walking for 30 minutes or whatever time you can manage is beneficial for your health.

✧ Avoid intense exercises in hot weather.

✧ Drink plenty of fluids during exercises.

✧ Make sure that your instructor or trainer or the fitness consultant is properly qualified and is aware of your pregnancy.

EXERCISES TO BE AVOIDED DURING PREGNANCY

✧ Exercises that have a risk of falling such as horse riding, skiing, skating, cycling, and gymnastics.

✧ Contact sports such as boxing, judo, kick boxing or martial arts.

✧ Scuba diving.

✧ Exercises over altitudes higher than 2500 metres above sea level. If you want to exercise at high altitudes, make sure you are properly acclimatised to that altitude before exercising.

OTHER EXERCISES TO BE DONE DURING PREGNANCY

✧ Stomach strengthening exercises.

✧ Pelvic tilt exercises.

✧ Pelvic floor strengthening exercises.

One very important thing to remember is that after 16 weeks of pregnancy, you should not lie flat on your back for prolonged periods as the weight of the baby presses on the main vein which carries blood of your lower body back to the heart and this could lead to fainting attacks.

Post Pregnancy Fitness

The first and foremost thing to consider is that pregnancy and post-pregnancy state is vastly different from one woman to another. Someone will be very fit before she conceived and someone might be overweight. Someone may develop complications during pregnancy like diabetes, pre-eclampsia or other conditions. Someone might have been advised bed rest. Someone might have a normal delivery or a C-section or the delivery might be complicated for any of the reasons.

All these factors should be taken into account when designing a fitness program for the new mom.

As a medical professional and as a trainer and a nutritionist, my first view would be that the new mom should try to achieve her fitness levels before pregnancy rather than trying to be a skinny bikini model.

Post-pregnancy fitness should actually begin during the pregnancy. It would be very difficult especially if you are having nausea, vomiting, lower back pain or swelling in the legs. You might have to go to the washroom many times during the night. You might not want to go for a full-fledged weight training or a Zumba session with the above complaints, but, remember one thing: TRY NOT TO GAIN EXCESSIVE WEIGHT DURING PREGNANCY.

The belief that 'A mother should eat for two' is completely wrong. This should not be an excuse for you to dig into pizza, cakes and donuts. Go for whole-grain items, lots of salads and proteins and good quality fats. Supplement yourself with calcium because a lot of calcium will be taken out of your bones if you are breast-feeding.

I suggest that you wait till you are completely healed before you enrol yourself into a full-fledged fitness program. You might have had an episiotomy or a C-section and it is always better to allow your body to completely heal first. Also, the pelvic joints are relaxed during pregnancy, so it is advisable not to indulge in heavy weight training sessions during this time. Light exercises will suffice. Go for group training sessions. If it is your second or third child, take your previous children with you to the garden and let them play while you walk around the park with your new born baby in the stroller. Before you know it, you would have walked about 30–45 minutes. This kind of activity will boost up your metabolism and will result in significant fat loss.

Remember one thing, being a mother does not give you an excuse to become over-weight. Try to achieve your pre-pregnancy fitness levels and you will see a remarkable change in your life. BE A SUPER MOM.

It is advisable to take the help of a medically qualified trainer in designing your fitness programs after delivery.

CHAPTER 50

FITNESS AFTER 50

50 years of life is the beginning of a glorious time when you have a rich experience of life behind you. You have time, you are successful in your career and you have a beautiful family with you. But, this is also the time when a person has all the lifestyle ailments like diabetes, hypertension, heart diseases and stroke. On the one hand, you are at the prime of your life and on the other hand, you have been bogged down by stress and other lifestyle disorders. Wouldn't you want to be physically fit and enjoy life at a time when you have the whole world at your disposal? Most of us will reply to this question in the affirmative. Let us see in this chapter what can be done so that you once again attain the youthful energy which you used to have 20 years ago.

Bodily changes after 50 years of age

There are certain changes in your body when you cross the 50 mark. You might not see this transition when you turn 40 but, at the age of 50, these changes are very marked. Let us see from a physiological point of view what exactly the changes are.

Your hormones especially the sex hormones decline with age. Now, from a fitness perspective, I am talking about two hormones mainly; those are testosterone and growth hormone. Testosterone is present in males as well as females. Both the sexes experience a decline of this hormone after the age of 30. This decline is more marked after 50 years of age. This hormone is associated with lean body mass especially muscle mass, bone strength and a general feeling of well-being. The immune system works better and there is a better recuperative ability of the body. This hormone is also associated with sexual drive in both the sexes. Similar is the growth hormone from the pituitary gland which helps in recovery and growth. Both these hormones are associated with fat burning. That is precisely the reason why so many youngsters eat junk food and still get away with it most of the time. Both these hormones are also associated with a general feeling of well-being.

Both these hormones decline very rapidly after the age of 40 years. There is a decrease of lean body mass as a result of decreased hormones and the metabolism becomes sluggish. Osteoporosis sets in the females earlier than the males after menopause. As there is a decrease in lean body mass, body fat starts to accumulate. There is a decrease in the feeling of well-being. Sexual drive wanes. The vitality and vigour is lost and a general sense of apathy sets in.

Other things to consider are decreased joint mobility and lax tendons and ligaments. There will be creaks and groans coming from various joints because of early arthritic changes, especially the shoulder, knee and spinal joints. Blood flow to the organs diminishes because of atherosclerotic changes in the arteries and at times, the function of some organs like the liver and kidneys are compromised.

By enumerating these points, I am not trying to say that you cannot be fit after 50 years of age. What I mean to say is that these points just have to be circumvented and the workout and dietary protocols modified to suit your needs.

FITNESS AFTER 50

The first thing to understand is that one should never be counting the calories burnt when exercising. If more calories are burnt, it usually indicates muscle loss and very rarely fat loss. Hence, cardio should never be the cornerstone of a fitness regime after the age of 50 years. Our aim is to gradually increase or to preserve the existing lean body mass, hence weight training is the answer after 50 years of age.

The foremost thing to do before prescribing a fitness regime to any person above the age of 50 years is to have a thorough medical examination and health check-up to rule out any potential ailments. The blood pressure and blood sugars should be checked and an electrocardiogram taken to know whether there is any problem with the blood supply to the heart or whether there are any rhythm disturbances. If there is any doubt, further investigations like echocardiography or treadmill stress test should be done. Liver and kidney parameters should be checked. If any abnormal values are detected, then they should either be corrected with diet, exercise or medications or your fitness prescription has to be worked around these abnormalities.

HOW WEIGHT TRAINING SHOULD BE PERFORMED

There should be an extensive phase of warm-up before any workout is begun. Every major joint of the body should be mobilised. Stretching in this age group should be done both before and after the workout.

While performing the sets, not using a barbell is a useful technique as there are lesser chances of injury, unless you are an experienced lifter with many years of experience in weight training. Certain compound exercises like bench press, military press, squats and deadlifts, if done with a barbell can make you injury-prone. If you are a novice in weight training, it is always advisable to start your training with dumbbells. Compound exercises should be performed with strict form and they should never be very heavy. You should stop a few repetitions before muscle failure. There is no reason why you should go beyond failure as described in the previous chapters as high intensity techniques are very taxing on the entire body systems. You start with light dumbbells and then gradually increase the weights. Weight train for about 3 days in a week and keep 3 days in a week for cardio.

Use isolation movements more. It is better to perform dumbbell lateral raises for your delts than wide grip barbell rows, which has a capacity to damage your shoulder joint. Triceps push downs are a better alternative to close grip bench press or dips.

If you are an experienced lifter who has been hitting the gym for several years, then there is no reason for you to change your schedule. You can continue lifting till a ripe old age.

Machines are your best friends now

The dictum of using free weights sounds good for young people. Free weights develop more muscles because your accessory muscles come into play. They lead to more muscular development. But, these same free weights also make you more prone to injury. When you have begun weight training after the age of 50 years, it would be safer for you to switch to machines from barbells. Dumbbells are still a safer alternative.

Nutrition

Your diet should be more of a clean diet with good amounts of proteins rather than going for those bulking and cutting diets advocated by trainers. Just make sure you do not resort to any extreme forms of dieting. Alcohol should be restricted to 1–2 pegs per week. If you are a diabetic or a hypertensive, your diet should be according to your medical condition.

No excuses should be there for not exercising at any age. Just a few aspects have to be modified and you can have a go at it. No age is exempt from fitness. Join a fitness program now under the guidance of a proper and experienced tutor and believe me, age will not be able to catch up with you.

CHAPTER 51

CARDIAC SURGERY AND FITNESS

I am a cardiac surgeon so, it is very obvious that I will be writing about this topic. But, the general principles outlined in this chapter can be applied to any post-operative patient.

This is yet another controversial topic from my bag, but, I speak what I think is logically correct and which I have tried out in many patients and clients. Many of you must be knowing people who have undergone heart surgery. Just ask them about their physical activity level. All of them will unanimously say that their doctor has advised them a little bit of aerobic activity such as walking or breathing exercises. But, look from the patient's point of view. Many patients who have undergone bypass surgery are 60+ years of age. They also want to live an active life and play with their grandchildren. They also want to do some gardening. They also want to be free to travel and lift their own luggage. In short, they don't want their life to be dependent on others. And we tell them exactly the opposite. We tell them to avoid strenuous work even though many years have passed after their surgery. Many people are made to believe that after their heart surgery, they should only be resting and living a retired life.

What I tell my patients is that cardiac surgery is not done so that they can retire. Only if my patients agree to live a really active life do I operate upon them. And believe me, most of my patients are so active that they can put most youngsters to shame.

Examine a cardiac patient a few months after he/she has undergone cardiac surgery. The person will have a shrunken chest with weak chest, back, shoulder and arm muscles. 'FROZEN SHOULDERS' in which there is a severe restriction of shoulder mobility in any range of motion is very commonly found. The reason is that they have never been taught the exercises for these body parts. All they are ever told is walking first on a flat surface and then, on an incline. The highest level of fitness activity advocated to them is climbing stairs. They are hammered with the idea that they should not be lifting anything for three-six months. It so happens that their muscles start to de-condition and shoulder mobility gets restricted. Then, they are not able to lift anything at all. The vicious circle!

You will find most post-operative patients with big tummies. This is obvious because the exercise they do is slow walking with their friends. If you analyse the 'healthy diet' prescribed by dieticians to them, you will find loads and loads of carbohydrates and fibres. The belly has to grow because metabolism will be at the lowest because of hypo-caloric diets and decreased lean body mass because of inactivity.

How should a post-operative cardiac patient be managed?

These patients have undergone a major surgical procedure. Their body is in a catabolic phase. What happens in catabolism? The stress hormones rise in the blood. Body tissues undergo breakdown. The surgical sites have to heal. Now, if you analyse the diets given to these patients, they are low calorie carbohydrate laden diets. Dieticians have this concept that body needs energy to heal at this stage, hence the increased carbohydrate load in the diet. The body needs proteins for healing the tissue and not carbohydrates. These patients are in the ICU and they are not undergoing any intense activity. Then, why the carbohydrates? These patients mobilise proteins from their stores that is skeletal muscles which undergo severe breakdown to supply amino acids and proteins to the healing surgical site. No wonder most of these patients look wasted after a few days stay in the hospital.

Let us analyse from a cardiac surgeon and a trainer-nutritionist's point of view how these patients should be managed. First of all, one thing should be clear to everyone that these patients are in a phase of very severe catabolism. They definitely require more proteins that their maintenance values and that also, a very high quality protein with high biological value. Most of these patients are diabetics. And they are at rest meaning they are not performing any intense activity in the ICU or in the wards. Hence, it can be safely assumed that they are in a basal resting state where most of the calories burnt will be from the fat stores. I would say that some quantities of good fats should be provided in the diet. And there should be no excuse about cholesterol in the fats. I have stated ample times that American Heart Association has removed cholesterol from the list of banned substances. It has been proved time and time again that there is no correlation between cholesterol and heart disease. So, a particular quantity of fats is very important in the diet of these patients as it provides energy in their basal state. Some amount of low glycemic carbohydrates should be given so that fats can be utilised as fuel because presence of carbohydrates are a must if fat is to be used as fuel. A good supplement of multivitamins and minerals especially zinc and calcium is very essential if the surgical site has to heal.

The idiocy of 'light' and 'heavy' diet

What exactly do people mean by a light diet? It implies that the food items which are given are digested easily and good motions are passed without any effort. Hence, the diets prescribed by dieticians to post-operative patients. My take on this is that prescribing wrong macro-nutrients under the pretext of easy digestibility is impermissible. Many proteins are available in the market like Whey proteins which are easily digested and can provide a very rich source of amino acids. Mind you, I am definitely not advocating the many protein formulations available in the pharmacy stores as most of them are laden with carbohydrates with very little protein in them.

Many of you might scoff at the idea of eating proteins post-operatively saying that they are not digestible during this time. Your gastric, intestinal and pancreatic juices which are stimulated by meals contain all the enzymes necessary for digestion of not only carbohydrates but also proteins and fats. And if the protein is fast digesting with good net digestibility and bioavailability, then why not consume it? And if you are so much concerned with stools, then take some fibres in your meals. Only eating carbohydrates is a very poor practice.

And there is nothing like 'light' and 'heavy food.' These terms are only used to connote the quantity of food taken in the meal. The meal should be light.

What physical training should be given to a cardiac patient?

Any bone fracture takes around 8 weeks to heal completely. We have to cut the breast bone to gain access to the heart. While closing the chest, stainless steel wires are used to bring the cut edges of the bone together. Since these patients are in an older age group and also have concomitant diseases like diabetes, blood pressure and osteoporosis, let us give them another month to heal their cut breast bone. After three months, bones are sufficiently united to take light weights. During these three months, the tissues need more than sufficient proteins, vitamins and minerals for complete recovery. It has been proved that resistance training will induce new bone formation at the sites where the exercising muscles are attached. New blood vessels will form at the site and the scar tissue which will be laid down at the operation site will certainly be very strong.

Resistance training and Cardiac Rehabilitation

Nowadays, many hospitals have a 'Department of Cardiac Rehabilitation' which is touted as a new marketing gimmick. What exactly is done in these departments? The physiotherapists make these patients undergo passive movements and some form of cardio like walking on the treadmill or cycling a stationary bike. Is performing light intensity exercise the only form of cardiac rehabilitation? Think again. These are very poor forms of fitness.

The muscles of the chest, back, shoulders and arms have remained inactive for a few months after cardiac surgery. They shrink (we call it 'atrophy' in medical terminology). These are the muscles which need to be strengthened and at the same time balanced. A program of weight training with gradual increase in resistance which balances opposite muscle groups like chest and back along with judicious amounts of cardio will slowly restore the muscles to their normal size and strength sufficiently so that these patients can live their lives in a normal way. They can even pick up their grandchildren and play with them and also lift their own luggage while travelling. Not a bad thing to re-achieve your life's vitality and vigour, isn't it?

CHAPTER 52
FITNESS SCENARIO IN INDIA

India is becoming the capital of lifestyle ailments in the world. Diseases like diabetes, hypertension, cardiac diseases and stroke are on a rise. Obesity has reached epidemic proportions and childhood obesity is increasing by leaps and bounds. There has been a sudden outcropping of gymnasiums and fitness centres all over the country but, fast food joints are springing up at a faster rate. There is a rat race in India to acquire a luxurious life in a short time and as a result, there has been total disregard for health. People are resorting to junk food because they just do not have the time to prepare a decent meal. Fitness is on a decline in this country.

Taking advantage of this scenario, there has been an outcropping of many fitness gurus many of whom are self-styled and uncertified. They resort to all sort of banned performance enhancing substances to build a lean and muscular physique and then, you find them preaching sermons on fitness and natural bodybuilding. In this era, the public is actually baffled because of the innumerable fitness websites and groups who attract more clients by offering fat loss packages at very cheap rates. Many Fad diet centres have come into the market, offering meal replacements many of which are nothing more than drinks without any authentic formulations. Many unqualified self-styled dieticians have jumped at the chance to offer their services to the hapless public by playing on their emotions. I see many dieticians advocating 'Ghar ka Khana' and 'Dadi Maa ka Khana' and diverting the minds of people by giving false information. If you really calculate the nutritional value of their diets it looks like junk. But, when someone appeals to your feelings of love towards your mother or grandmother, you tend to get swayed by such statements.

The gym and trainers

Countless people pay their full annual fees in the gym. They enter the gym with lots of hopes and enthusiasm. But, their enthusiasm soon wanes when there is no result. After all, how many trainers have the requisite knowledge of the human body, its biochemistry, metabolism and the hormonal responses to exercise? Nowadays, anyone and everyone becomes a trainer. I have seen countless candidates joining the gym as a trainer and then, learning the exercises from their seniors. It is like one blind man leading another blind man; both will fall in the ditch. It is not only the exercises that matter but, the correct prescription of exercises based on the body habitus, lifestyle and goals of the client that will pave the way for his/her transformation. It seems that there is no lack of trainers in this country but, what India needs is qualified trainers with a flair for fitness, who see the fitness field more as a passion whose services have to be delivered in an exemplary fashion.

Gyms and the society

Most people in our Indian society have a lot of apprehension when it comes to the gym. When asked the reason, no one is able to pinpoint the exact cause. People are just scared to go to the gym. I cannot decipher the reason. One lame excuse every client gives is when we will lose weight and then, leave the gym, we will regain what we have lost. My answer to this is why would you leave the gym? There are many stupid excuses heard but, they are not worth mentioning here. Just take this statement at its face value that given a chance, people do not want to join the gym. Maybe, it's plain laziness. Or maybe people would rather want to spend money on a hospital bed rather than a fitness plan. The reasons are best known to them.

Health vs. Medical, Pharma and the Food industry

There is a big chasm in the fitness scenario in India with health on one side and the medical, pharma and food industry on the other. There seems to be an all-out war. The medical industry is being directed by the pharma industry. It has been amply proved many times that there is no correlation between cholesterol and heart disease. There is no such thing as good cholesterol and bad cholesterol. And I am not talking through my hat. I am quoting the newest guidelines from the American Heart Association. I bet all the cardiologists and physicians must have read this, but who cares. Newer and newer cholesterol lowering drugs are introduced in the market almost every year. And the pharma industry touts clinical research about those drugs which are self-sponsored. Incentives are given to the doctors who defy all logic and give those medicines to people even if they have normal lipid levels. And I am a cardiac surgeon who deals with blockages in the arteries on a daily basis, and I want to shout from the roof tops and say that cholesterol lowering agents have very little value. More than 90% of your body's cholesterol is produced by your own liver. Trying to suppress your normal cholesterol production using unnatural means will cause more harm than good. And I want the advocates of these medicines to please find out what is the importance of cholesterol in the body. Simple biochemistry learnt in the first year of medical college, isn't it!

Hypothyroidism has become a business nowadays. Thyroid hormones are being prescribed on the slightest pretext. The threshold for thyroid hormone replacement therapy has become very low. If you see the initial reports of the so-called hypothyroid patients, you will find isolated raised TSH levels. The first and foremost cause of this blood picture is 'Iodine Deficiency.' How many times has any effort been made to determine this cause? Never, and I mean NEVER. Thyroid gland is a burner and pituitary gland is a thermostat. By giving thyroid hormone replacement, you are stifling the burner and shutting off the thermostat at the same time. What logic! It is not that these mistakes are done wilfully. It is because as doctors, we have never paid much attention to biochemistry or nutrition. These subjects should be made compulsory in the medical curriculum and the certifications in these courses have to be updated on a yearly basis. Only then you will see good quality prevention.

My simple advice to all the dieticians: Nutritional science goes much beyond starvation diets. Healthy diets just do not mean giving diets of low glycemic index carbohydrates. Even correct proportions of proteins, fats, vitamins and minerals and how they are mixed in the diet have to be calculated. Learn to calculate diets based on the patient's various parameters. There cannot be a cut/copy-paste diet for everyone. Each individual is unique and the diet cannot be the same for everyone. Please try to go beyond the RDA values for macronutrients because these values are for the general population so that they can survive without exhibiting the symptoms and signs of any nutritional deficiency. The PDI values that are necessary for optimum fitness of people are much higher than the RDA values.

Body builders in India

Bodybuilding is supposed to be a costly sport. Many bodybuilders belong to the lower socio-economic strata of the society. It so happens that in order to pursue their passion, much of their income is being spent on their own diet and supplementation. Their families live frugally because there is hardly any money left to feed the other members. Many bodybuilders have broken homes as a result. Body building does not mean going to the gym once daily and then, forgetting about it. Body building is a 24 hours' passion – eating on time, sleeping on time, very poor social life etc. Compare bodybuilding in the western world with the sport in India. Where do you think we stand? I am not commenting about the quality of bodybuilders here. We have some of the best bodybuilders with the finest genetics, but the only reason why they fall short when they rub shoulders with the big guys in competitions like Mr. Universe and Mr. Olympia is because the western bodybuilders are sponsored bodybuilders. They have the best of trainers and the best of nutritionists to design their workouts and diet plans. Their diets and supplements are all sponsored, so all they do is concentrate on bodybuilding. Bodybuilding is an exact science and not just hoisting weights and eating protein. An average Indian bodybuilder has to run from pillar to post and beg for sponsorships. Many times they are told that unless they win a competition, they are not eligible for sponsorships. Imagine the mind of a bodybuilder. He trains throughout the year and sacrifices a lot of things in pursuit of that trophy which will give him a name in history. There can be only one winner. But, that does not mean that the other athletes have not given their worth. Each has worked as hard as the next guy. And when he does not get the prize, he just shrugs off his defeat and starts preparing for the next year with full enthusiasm. How do you expect him to be worrying all the time about where the meals and supplementation for the next month are going to come from and still expect him to win laurels for the country? This country has to wake up and recognise bodybuilding as a sport and give its bodybuilders their due.

Other sports in India

It is not only bodybuilding but many other sports that need recognition from the Indian public and government. India should now realise the fact that cricket is not the only sport in this country. Equal weightage should be given to other sports like badminton, football, hockey and many others. Thanks to some movies which have brought wrestling into the limelight. Many gold medallists in India are living anonymous lives. No one cares, not even the government. Seeing the pathetic state of many of the athletes, parents do not want their children to be sports persons. Plus, our dietary habits leave much to chance that the athlete will bring a medal for the country. Let the government recognise not only the established athletes but also the potential ones so that even our future is as good. Sponsorships and encouragement will go a long way in putting India on the sports map.

Fitness is last on an Indian's list

India is a strange country. Many Indians would rather spend lakhs of rupees on treating diseases rather than a few thousand on fitness. Why this sorry state of affairs exists is beyond the scope of anyone's comprehension. Maybe, there is not correct guidance in this country or maybe there are many charlatans masquerading as fitness gurus so that the Indian public is sceptical about spending their hard-earned money on them. The reasons may be numerous. I have seen people spending crores of rupees on weddings but, when they have to spend a few thousand on their fitness, they withdraw their hand. Is it laziness? Do they feel that why should they go to slog in the gym for an hour a day when they can sleep during that time or make a few more bucks? Life in India is very stressful, but then so is everywhere. No excuse is permissible for not exercising and living a healthy life.

CLOSING STATEMENTS

Through this book, I have tried to shed light on many aspects of fitness and medicine. I am a practising Cardiac Surgeon and I am very proud of that. But, I am more proud of the fact that I have not yet sacrificed my faculty of logical thinking to the whims of the Pharma Industry and 'Bro-Science.' Whatever is there in this book is based on what I have learnt about the anatomy, physiology and biochemistry of the human body in my first year of medical college, my certifications as a sports nutritionist and as an advanced master trainer and of course, detailed research on nutrition and exercise science. I have managed more than 1200 fitness clients till now (over and above my thousands of patients who underwent cardiac surgery by my hands) with outstanding and dramatic results. My advice to all of you who have taken the pains to read this book is that by now, you would have understood the importance of nutrition and exercise in your life. Let all of you make a pledge that today is the first day of the rest of your life. There is one and only one thing that truly belongs to you and that is your own body. Your body is your place of worship. Take care of it. Keep it clean and healthy. For even if you lose everything, your body will always remain with you till your last breath.

I wish you all a long and 'Scienti-fit' life.

Dependably Yours

Dr. Kalpesh Malik MBBS, MS (Gen surgery), M.Ch. (CVTS)

Senior Cardio-Vascular and Thoracic Surgeon

Master trainer from International Federation of Body building.

Sports Nutritionist from International Sports Sciences Association.

Founder and Director of THE SCIENTIFIT HEALTHCARE AND WELLNESS SERVICES.